Lecture Notes in Computer Science 6689

Russell H. Taylor   Guang-Zhong Yang (Eds.)

Information Processing in Computer-Assisted Interventions

Second International Conference, IPCAI 2011
Berlin, Germany, June 22, 2011
Proceedings

Springer

Volume Editors

Russell H. Taylor
The Johns Hopkins University
Dept. of Computer Science
MD 21218, Baltimore, USA
E-mail: rht@jhu.edu

Guang-Zhong Yang
Imperial College London
Department of Computing
London, SW7 2BZ, UK
E-mail: g.z.yang@imperial.ac.uk

ISSN 0302-9743 e-ISSN 1611-3349
ISBN 978-3-642-21503-2 ISBN 978-3-642-21504-9 (eBook)
DOI 10.1007/978-3-642-21504-9
Springer Heidelberg Dordrecht London New York

Library of Congress Control Number: 2011929043

CR Subject Classification (1998): I.6, I.4-5, J.3, I.2.10, I.2.9

LNCS Sublibrary: SL 6 – Image Processing, Computer Vision, Pattern Recognition, and Graphics

Typesetting: Camera-ready by author, data conversion by Scientific Publishing Services, Chennai, India

Printed on acid-free paper

Springer is part of Springer Science+Business Media (www.springer.com)

Preface

In the coming decades, information technology will have as profound an effect on interventional medicine as it has had on manufacturing, transportation, and many other segments of our society. Over the next 20 years, it will be possible to combine all pertinent information about an individual patient (including images, clinical records, lab results, genetics, medical history and other data) into a consistent representation of the patient. Powerful computational tools will help human physicians to diagnose the patient's condition, evaluate treatment options, and optimize a patient-specific treatment plan. During treatment, all of this information will be registered to the patient and updated with intraoperative images and sensors. Robotic devices, visualization aids, and other computer-based systems will assist clinicians in ensuring that the plan is executed accurately and safely. The patient's condition will be monitored both during the intervention and post-operatively to assess the efficacy of therapy and guide further treatment, again combining all available data on the patient with subject-specific models describing likely outcomes and complications.

The focus of the Information Processing and Computer-Assisted Intervention (IPCAI) Conferences is the use of information technology in interventional medicine, including real-time modeling and analysis, technology, human–machine interfaces, and systems associated with operating rooms and interventional suites. It also covers the overall information flow associated with intervention planning, execution, follow-up, and outcome analysis, as well as training and skill assessment for such procedures. The goal is to provide a venue for presentation and in-depth discussion of the latest work in the field.

This volume contains the proceedings of the Second IPCAI Conference, following an extremely successful first meeting held in Geneva, Switzerland, on June 23, 2010. The organizers' original intention had been to hold IPCAI every other year, but further discussions with many of our colleagues within the field convinced us that an annual meeting of IPCAI would serve a valuable purpose.

This year, despite a late start, we received 29 full paper submissions (11 from Europe, 15 from North America, and 3 from elsewhere). These submissions were reviewed by a total of 49 external reviewers, coordinated by 6 Program Committee members. A "primary" and "secondary" Program Committee member was assigned to each paper, and each paper received at least three reviews. Authors were given the chance to respond to the reviews before final decisions were made. In some cases, acceptances were made conditional on specific requested changes and re-verification by the program committee. This process resulted in 17 very high quality accepted papers. In the final program, eight papers were presented and discussed in traditional platform presentations and the other nine were presented in an "interactive" session consisting of short 5-minute platform presentations and an extended poster session. This format was very productive in IPCAI 2010 and was even more so this year.

In closing, we would like to thank all the authors who submitted their papers to IPCAI for their conscientious efforts in responding to the reviews. We also thank the reviewers who provided high-quality reviews, which are very helpful to all authors, and the Program Committee members who gave so generously of their time.

June 2011

Russell Taylor
Guang-Zhong Yang

Organization

Executive Committee

Program Chairs

Russell Taylor	JHU, USA
Guang-Zhong Yang	Imperial College, UK

Area Chairs

Purang Abolmaesoumi	UBC, Canada
Kevin Cleary	DC Children's Hospital, USA
Dave Hawkes	UCL, UK
Thomas Langø	SINTEF, Norway
Tim Salcudean	UBC, Canada
Ichiro Sakuma	University of Tokyo, Japan

General Chair

Nassir Navab	CAMP/TUM, Germany

Publication Chair

Pierre Jannin	INRIA/INSERM, Rennes, France

Financial Chair

Leo Joskowicz	Hebrew University, Israel

Panel Chair

Kensaku Mori	Nagoya University, Japan

Local Organization Chair

Stefanie Demirci	CAMP/TUM, Germany

Publicity Chair

Martin Horn	CAMP/TU Munich, Germany

Scientific Review Committee

Systems, Software, and Validation

Yoshinobu Sato	Osaka, Japan
Luc Soler	IRCAD, France
Noby Hata	BWH, USA
Kirby Vosburgh	MGH, USA
Wolfgang Birkfellner	University of Vienna, Austria
Lutz Nolte	University of Bern, Switzerland
Randy Ellis	Queens University, Canada

Interventional Robotics and Navigation

Jocelyne Troccaz	TIMC /CNRS, France
Gabor Fichtinger	Queens University, Canada
Brian Davies	Imperial College, London, UK
Koji Ikuta	Nagoya, Japan
Kiyoyuki Chinzei	Tsukuba, Japan
Lena Maier-Hein	DKFZ, Germany

Surgical Planning, Simulation, and Advanced Intra-Op Visualization

Terry Peters	London, Canada
Gábor Székely	ETH, Switzerland
Hervé Delingette	INRIA, France
Ken Masamune	Tokyo, Japan
Sebastien Ourselin	London, UK

Interventional Imaging

Alison Noble	Oxford, UK
Emad Boctor	JHU, USA
Ali Kamen	SCR, USA
Joachim Hornegger	Erlangen, Germany
Pierre Hellier	Rennes, France
Ramtin Shams	ANU, Australia
Guoyan Zheng	Bern, Switzerland

Cognition, Modeling and Context Awareness

Louis Collins	BIC, Canada
Benoit Dawant	Vanderbilt, USA
Greg Hager	JHU, USA
Hayit Greenspan	Tel Aviv University, Israel
Peter Kazanzides	JHU, USA

Industrial Liaisons

Wolfgang Wein	White Lion Tech. GmbH, Germany
Ameet Jain	Philips, USA
Tom Vercauteren	Mauna Kea, France
Simon DiMaio	Intuitive Surgical, USA
Joerg Traub	SurgicEye, Germany
Leslie Holton	Medtronic, USA

Reviewers

Purang Abolmaesumi
Ahmad Ahmadi
Wolfgang Birkfellner
Emad Boctor
Kiyoyuki Chinzei
Kevin Cleary
Louis Collins
Benoit Dawant
Herve Delingette
Randy Ellis
Aron Fenster
Gabor Fichtinger
Penney Graeme
Noby Hata
Dave Hawkes
Pierre Hellier
Joachim Hornegger
Pierre Jannin
Leo Joskowicz
Ali Kamen
Peter Kazanzides
Thomas Lango
Andras Lasso
Sulin Lee
Frank Lindseth
Lena Maier-Hein
Ken Masamune
Jamie McClelland
Kensaku Mori
Sebastien Muller
Yukitaka Nimura
Alison Noble
Lutz Nolte
Sebastien Ourselin
Nicolas Padoy
Terry Peters
Tobias Reichl
Ingerid Reinertsen
Robert Rohling
Ichiro Sakuma
Tim Salcudean
Yoshinobu Sato
Tormod Selbekk
Luc Soler
Ole Solheim
Raphael Sznitman
Russ Taylor
Jocelyne Troccaz
Tom Vercauteren
Kirby Vosburgh
Wolfgang Wein
Ziv Yaniv

Table of Contents

Surgical Planning, Simulation, and Guidance

The Tumor Therapy Manager – Design, Refinement and Clinical Use of a Software Product for ENT Surgery Planning and Documentation 1
Ivo Rössling, Jana Dornheim, Lars Dornheim, Andreas Boehm, and Bernhard Preim

An Image-Guided Surgery System to Aid Endovascular Treatment of Complex Aortic Aneurysms: Description and Initial Clinical Experience 13
Graeme Penney, Andreas Varnavas, Neville Dastur, and Tom Carrell

OR Specific Domain Model for Usability Evaluations of Intra-operative Systems 25
Ali Bigdelou, Tobias Sterner, Stefan Wiesner, Thomas Wendler, Florian Matthes, and Nassir Navab

A Multi-view Active Contour Method for Bone Cement Reconstruction from C-Arm X-Ray Images 36
Blake C. Lucas, Yoshito Otake, Mehran Armand, and Russell H. Taylor

Biomechanically Constrained Groupwise Statistical Shape Model to Ultrasound Registration of the Lumbar Spine 47
Siavash Khallaghi, Parvin Mousavi, Dan Borschneck, Gabor Fichtinger, and Purang Abolmaesumi

Visual Tracking of Surgical Tools for Proximity Detection in Retinal Surgery 55
Rogério Richa, Marcin Balicki, Eric Meisner, Raphael Sznitman, Russell Taylor, and Gregory Hager

Medical Robotics, Instrumentation, and Modelling

DOF Minimization for Optimized Shape Control under Active Constraints for a Hyper-redundant Flexible Robot 67
Valentina Vitiello, Ka-Wai Kwok, Christopher Payne, and Guang-Zhong Yang

A Robotic System for Intra-operative Trans-Rectal Ultrasound and Ultrasound Elastography in Radical Prostatectomy 79
Troy Adebar, Septimiu Salcudean, Sara Mahdavi, Mehdi Moradi, Christopher Nguan, and Larry Goldenberg

Hand-Held Force Magnifier for Surgical Instruments 90
George Stetten, Bing Wu, Roberta Klatzky, John Galeotti, Mel Siegel, Randy Lee, Francis Mah, Andrew Eller, Joel Schuman, and Ralph Hollis

PS-GANS: A Patient-Specific, Gravity Assisted Navigation System for Acetabular Cup Placement 101
Guoyan Zheng, Santiago Echeverri, Weiguo Xie, and Lutz-Peter Nolte

Correlating Clinical Scores with Anatomical Electrodes Locations for Assessing Deep Brain Stimulation 113
Florent Lalys, Claire Haegelen, Alexandre Abadie, and Pierre Jannin

Intra-operative "Pick-Up" Ultrasound for Robot Assisted Surgery with Vessel Extraction and Registration: A Feasibility Study 122
Caitlin Schneider, Julian Guerrero, Christopher Nguan, Robert Rohling, and Septimiu Salcudean

Abdominal Navigation and Visualization

Constrained 2-D/3-D Registration for Motion Compensation in AFib Ablation Procedures 133
Alexander Brost, Andreas Wimmer, Rui Liao, Joachim Hornegger, and Norbert Strobel

Image-Based Automatic Ablation Point Tagging System with Motion Correction for Cardiac Ablation Procedures 145
YingLiang Ma, Gang Gao, Geert Gijsbers, C. Aldo Rinaldi, Jaswinder Gill, Reza Razavi, and Kawal S. Rhode

Passive Single Marker Tracking for Organ Motion and Deformation Detection in Open Liver Surgery 156
Thiago Oliveira-Santos, Matthias Peterhans, Simon Hofmann, and Stefan Weber

Interventional Imaging

Improved Neuronavigation through Integration of Intraoperative Anatomical and Diffusion Images in an Interventional MRI Suite 168
Pankaj Daga, Gavin Winston, Marc Modat, M. Jorge Cardoso, Mark White, Laura Mancini, Andrew W. McEvoy, John Thornton, Caroline Micallef, Tarek Yousry, David Hawkes, John S. Duncan, and Sebastien Ourselin

Panorama Ultrasound for Guiding Epidural Anesthesia: A Feasibility Study 179
Hedyeh Rafii-Tari, Purang Abolmaesumi, and Robert Rohling

Author Index 191

The Tumor Therapy Manager – Design, Refinement and Clinical Use of a Software Product for ENT Surgery Planning and Documentation

Ivo Rössling[1], Jana Dornheim[2], Lars Dornheim[2], Andreas Boehm[3], and Bernhard Preim[1]

[1] Otto-von-Guericke University, Faculty of Computer Science, Department of Simulation and Graphics, Magdeburg, Germany
{ivo.roessling,bernhard.preim}@ovgu.de
[2] Dornheim Medical Images GmbH, Magdeburg, Germany
{jana,lars}@dornheim-medical-images.de
[3] University of Leipzig, Medical Faculty, Germany
andreas.boehm@medizin.uni-leipzig.de

Abstract. The treatment of patients with head and neck cancers is a demanding medical field, due to the compact anatomy and complex functionality of the affected region. The planning process comprises issues regarding risk and applicability of intervention, extent of surgical removal, and the choice of appropriate access to the pathology. Required clinical information are obtained from different examinations, ranging from external visual and palpatory inspection, over preoperative panendoscopy and biopsy histology to radiological imaging.

The surgeon needs to process all available information in mind and virtually compile a mental patient model of the target anatomy. 3D visualizations of tomographic data may improve perception of spatial relationships. However, discussions with clinical practicians reveal that parameterization of advanced visual effects tend to be cumbersome and resulting visualizations are often too complex and not dedicated to specific diagnostic or treatment planning questions. Moreover, they will add valuable alternative views, but cannot replace all the other diagnostic sources.

We describe long-term experiences on developing and refining a software for ENT surgery planning and documentation. Regarding 3D visualizations, it turns out to be superior to generate sequences of rather simple 3D views directly supporting specific treatment questions, instead of presenting many anatomic structures simultaneously. Developing software for clinical practice thereby benefits from a thorough understanding of the target scenarios and the "visual questions" they raise. The second focus is on the seamless integration of the different diagnostic modalities, findings, and therapy decisions into a common electronic document. We report on the actual clinical use of the system and discuss how it fits into the surgical planning workflow.

Keywords: ENT, HNSCC, tomography, panendoscopy, segmentation, CAD, surgery planning, documentation.

R.H. Taylor and G.-Z. Yang (Eds.): IPCAI 2011, LNCS 6689, pp. 1–12, 2011.

1 Introduction

The treatment of patients with head and neck cancers is more and more challenging in the regard of raising therapeutic alternatives and a multidisciplinary approach. Initial diagnostics is thereby considerably gaining in importance, not least due the growing multitude of chemo-therapeutic options – in addition to or as replacement for surgical interventions – that may involve potentially significant cost increases (medicament costs for chemotherapy of up to 40.000 EUR per patient). However, even continuously improving precision and quality of pretherapeutic imaging does not generally suffice to sound all therapeutic means exhaustively.

This in particular applies for interventional measures in ENT surgery. Complexity in anatomy of the head and neck here still results in difficulties in the preoperative planning even for well experienced surgeons. Tomography data can help identifying abnormalities, but do not always entirely reveal the overall picture of spatial relations in three-dimensional space, and not all kinds of malignant tissue may be directly visible based on CT or MR imaging. Additional findings are obtained via classical visual and palpatory inspection, in particular panendoscopy. At present, the surgeon is obligated to process all available information in mind and virtually compile a mental patient model of the target anatomy, including blood vessels, nerve supply, muscles and tendons, and more.

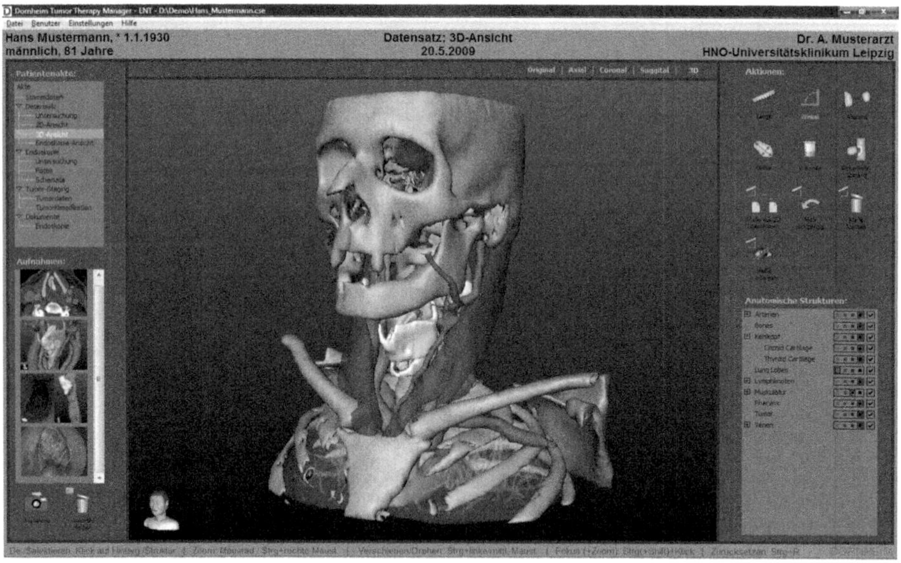

Fig. 1. Patient-individual neck anatomy as derived from CT data, shown in the TTM. Click left to activate the embedded PDF3d model, then right click for context menu. (Requires Adobe Acrobat Reader 7.0 or newer. Best viewed in fullscreen multimedia mode. Structure visibilities changeable. Predefined views result from dynamic snapshots created by TTM user).

The planning process comprises decisions on issues, such as applicability of an intervention, extent of surgical removal, selection of an appropriate access to the pathology, and exploration of adjacent anatomic structures to evaluate the interventional risk. Due to the compact anatomy and complex functionality of the affected region, adherence of oncologically sufficient safety distances thereby comes for the price of the potential risk of functional losses.

Facing this issue, 3D visualizations of the neck anatomy (Fig. 1) can provide a real added value, ranging from fast overview to in-depth visual-spatial exploration. Moreover, if they were obtained by segmentation of the relevant target structures, the corresponding 3D representations carry geometric information that can be used to generate visualizations directly supporting specific diagnostic or treatment planning questions, such as the volume or diameter of a tumor, its distance to a nearby risk structure, the existence of potential infiltrations, etc. The geometry may also be used for automatic semantic reasoning, e. g. in the context of tumor staging. Re-using available information is in general a beneficial objective. In fact, the combination of original tomography data, the derived 3D visualizations and the inclusion of further modalities and non-radiological information like endoscopic examinations, palpatory findings and histological results provide the best means to complete the surgeon's mental model and to support him in diagnostics, therapy planning, and documentation.

2 Project Background

To develop image analysis and visualization algorithms and to integrate them into a dedicated software assistant for the above mentioned and related questions was the goal of two sequential national research projects, starting in 2004 and lasting five years in total. Research was focussed on automatic segmentation of relevant structures, e.g. lymph nodes [1] and blood vessels [2] and advanced visualization of these structures, e.g. by cut-away views for emphasizing lymph nodes [3] and careful combinations of slicebased and 3D visualizations [4].

Two research prototypes, the NeckSegmenter for segmentation and the NeckSurgeryPlanner [5] for interactive exploration and surgery planning were developed and used in clinical practice since 2006. The clinical partners started to present these systems first internally, e.g. at the tumorboard, and later at their workshops and conferences [6,7] leading to additional and generally positive feedback. Based on this feedback, interest from a leading industry supplier, and the continuous support of the clinical partners, a spin-off company, Dornheim Medical Images, was founded in early 2008 in order to transform the prototypes in product quality software (Dornheim TumorTherapyManager) ready for market and clinical practice.

3 In-Depth Task Analysis

As a major prerequisite for re-developing a research prototype into a practical tool for broad real world use, we entered again in a stage of in-depth task

analysis. While in the research project, a trade-off between scientifically interesting questions and real needs was required, a rigorous analysis of tasks, preferences and priorities was necessary for the actual clinical use. This analysis was accomplished as a larger set of interviews at the ENT department in Leipzig as well as observations of clinical processes including surgery.
This analysis was focussed on an understanding of:

1. individual surgical planning and preoperative decisions,
2. integration of information from multiple examinations,
3. collaborative treatment planning and tumor boards,
4. patient consultation, and
5. documentation.

To represent the results, informal scenario descriptions [8] have been created, discussed, refined, and verified by discussing them with the clinical experts. These scenarios describe different clinical cases, all examinations which are accomplished to come to a diagnosis, the planning process and the post-operative situation. Special care was necessary to cover a representative set of different diseases (different with respect to number and size of metastasis, location of metastasis, infiltration of risk structures). A few examples, related to selected issues of the list above, might highlight this process.

3D Understanding. The review and quantification of spatial relationships turned out to be crucial for preoperative risk assessment and access planning. This calls for detailled 3D understanding of the anatomical setting (Figs. 2 and 3) which cannot be fully provided by slice-based viewing of tomography data (Fig. 2, left).

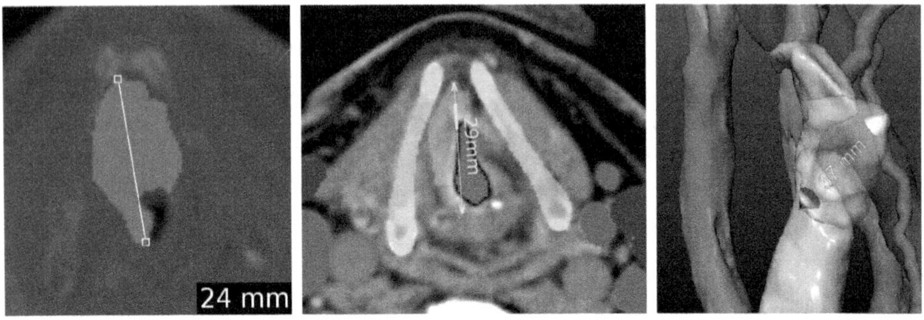

Fig. 2. Measurement of tumor diameter in a real clinical case. *Left*: The common practice of measuring by hand in selected axial CT slices suggested a maximum extent of 24mm. *Middle*: Support for slice-spanning manual measurements (intersection with the current slice is painted bold) provides means for assessing also the third dimension. However, finding the actual extreme points can be tedious. *Right*: If segmentations are at hand, the diameter can be derived fully-automatically. The tumor extent turned out to be more than 50% larger. The resulting measure can be visualized in 2d as a slice-spanning distance. A 3D scene, however, provides better perception of overall spatial relationships.

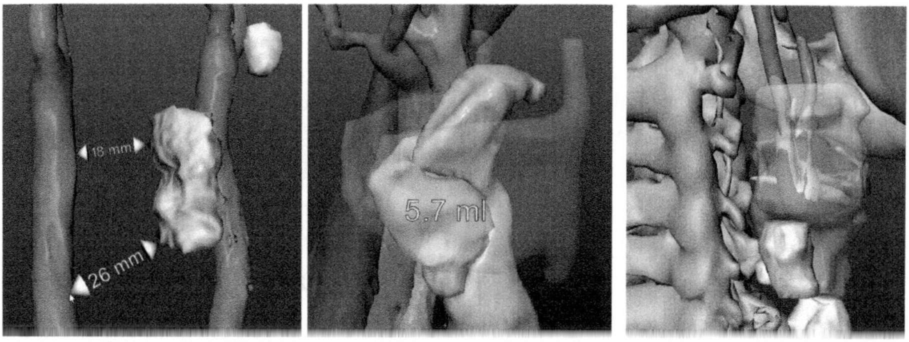

Fig. 3. 3D visualizations supporting specific treatment questions. *Left*: According to the given segmentations, the effective minimum distance between tumor and arteria carotis is 18mm. In case this measure is not expressive enough, the clinician can also fix the tumor and interactively discover the blood vessel's surface, retrieving the perpendicular to the malignant tissue in real-time. *Middle*: Volumetry for a tumor occupying the space between cricoid and thyroid cartilage and pharynx. *Right*: Color-coding of safety distance violation allows to assess contact and infiltration areas that are usually occluded. The figure shows arteria carotis color-coded w. r. t. the partially enclosing tumor and two violation levels (*yellow*=3mm or closer, *strong red*=1mm or closer).

Infiltrations. It turned out that infiltrations of anatomic structures by a tumor are investigated in detail w. r. t. their likelihood and extent. Thus, dedicated visualizations are desired containing just the risk structure, the tumor and the possible infiltration area (see Fig. 3 and the two user-captured views for thyroid cartilage within the interactive scene in Fig. 1).

Volumetry. Besides its extent and distance to or infiltration of nearby risk structures, the volume taken up by malignant tissue (Fig. 3, middle) crucially determines possible therapy options.

Panendoscopic Findings. Besides CT or MRI, endoscopic interventions are the most important source of information relevant for ENT surgical decisions. The surgeon investigates possible tumors using optical view and touch sense. Then, special sheets of paper with pre-printed schematic drawings of the neck anatomy are used to annotate the findings by hand (Fig. 7). The task analysis clearly revealed a need for integrating this information with the electronic documentation and the findings from CT data.

Documentation. For medical doctors in general, and for surgeons in particular, a careful documentation of diagnostic information, treatment decisions and patient consultation is essential because of juristic reasons and of the account with social insurance. Such bureaucratic tasks are time-consuming and annoying for the surgeons. Thus, any support which shortens the documentation is highly welcome (Figs. 6 and 7).

4 The Tumor Therapy Manager

The whole development of the TumorTherapyManager (TTM) was guided by an understanding of the clinical workflow and resulted in a modular design of corresponding components. Grouped around a central patient record, the basic workflow is made up by set of examinations, potential tumor staging, and the generation of documents.

Tomography. Each examination covers basic examination information, acquired imaging data, resulting findings and therapy options. For modalities CT and MRT, the integrated DICOM-Viewer offers direct slice-based exploration of tomography data. If segmentations are available, their voxel masks can be selectively overlayed to the dataset. Apart from that, the TTM provides a 3D visualization of the corresponding surfaces. A new unified measurement

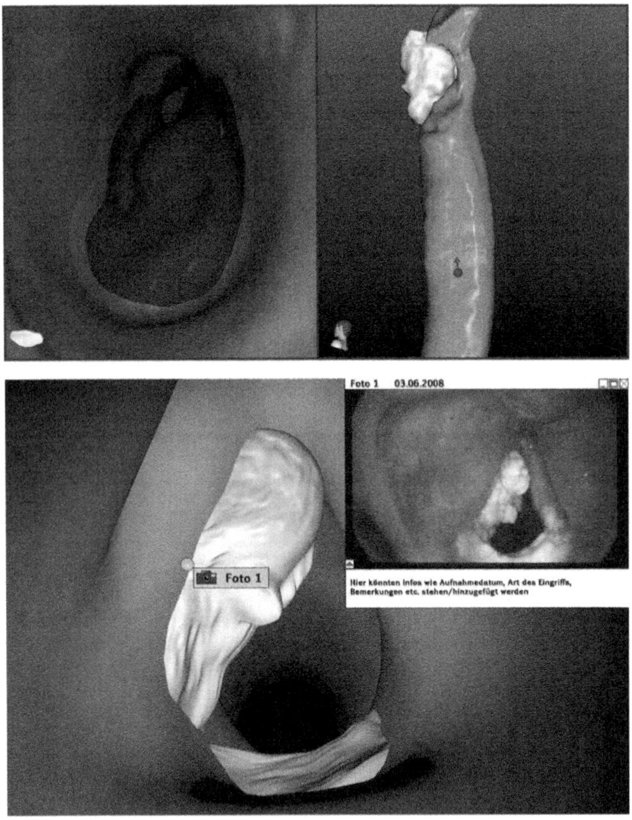

Fig. 4. *Top:* Virtual endoscopy and 3D context in side-by-side view. *Left:* Safety distance colorization of inner pharynx surface reveals outside contact areas. *Right:* Red glyph indicates view position and direction. A glass-like effect provides better visual perception than simple transparency. *Bottom:* For a tumor grown through the pharynx wall, a photo of the real intervention is attached to the corresponding position.

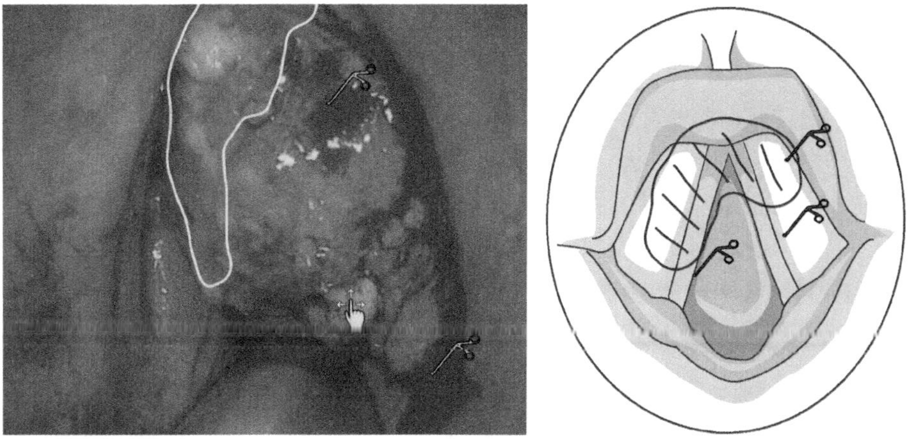

Fig. 5. The panendoscopy module offers easy annotation functionality. *Left:* An endoscopy photo is enriched with a line indicating the alleged tumor boundary, with markers depicting biopsy positions and with a hint concerning tissue movability. *Right:* A schematic pictogram is annotated with the affected area and biopsy positions.

approach [9] was implemented, capable of covering a variety of different distance based 3D measures (shortest distance, largest diameter, infiltration boundary, safety margins, etc.) for most different kinds of input (manual points, structures, groups, computed geometries like center points, skeletons, etc.). For optimal usability, the current view can freely be switched (axial, sagittal, coronal, 3D) during the running measurement.

For specific structures (e. g., the respiratory tract) an additional virtual endoscopy is provided that allows closer examination of the interior. Although visualizations generated from tomography data like CT or MRT cannot reflect the exact surface texture, an added value is given by revealing outside contact areas or combining virtual view with real photos (Fig. 4).

Panendoscopy. Real endoscopy itself is granted its own modality. Its imaging data consists of photos acquired during endoscopic examination and schematic drawings. For both types of pictures a user-friendly annotation system is provided – with freehand drawings, textual labels, and simple icons depicting important areas, (im)movable tissue or biopsy positions. Using the latter feature during endoscopy allows for unambiguous identification of biopsies by capturing id and position (usually a potential source of error). Besides visual evidence, these annotation features offer an easy way for incorporating also non-visual perceptions such as palpatory findings (Fig. 5).

Tumor Staging. The tumor staging module provides form-based support for collecting tumor data and conducting a classification. For maximum support of the user, the application is capable of suggesting values whenever the information can be derived from the segmented geometries (Fig. 6). That is, for the tumor

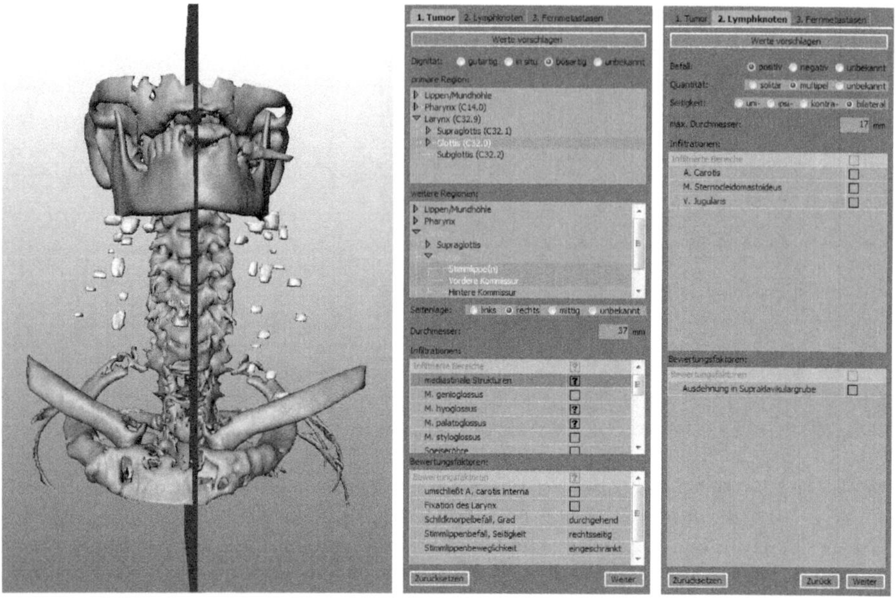

Fig. 6. Deriving information from the segmented geometries. *Left:* Based on a computed estimation of the midsagittal plane, sideness and laterality can be determined fully-automatically. *Middle & Right*: Suggested values (*blue*) for e. g. extent, quantity, sideness, and laterality ease up the process of tumor staging. *Middle:* The integrated TNM-classifier computes an objectively correct classification for the entered data and alerts in case of missing information.

and all malignant-marked lymph nodes, extent and quantity can be computed easily. Based on a computed estimate of the midsagittal plane (see [10]), also sideness and laterality can be determined fully-automatically.

Moreover, a complete TNM classifier for ENT tumors has been implemented to ensure that all relevant data has been gathered and that (based on the expert's subjective assessment) the resulting TNM classification is correct according to the official rules of AJCC and UICC [11,12]

Documentation. For any modality, snapshots of the current view (Fig. 1, left bar) can be made for the purpose of documentation. Besides plain screenshots, the 3D views also offer the possibility for capturing individual states of the scene and collecting them in an interactive 3D model (Fig. 1), thereby providing enhanced means for documentation and exchange of opinions (e. g. tumor board).

The TTM's documentation module finally allows for incorporating the available information into documents of pre-defined format (Fig. 7). Since LaTeX is used as generator, the layout is freely user-definable and can in particular be branded to the individual institution. At present, a template for the panendoscopy document sheet of the ENT department in Leipzig has been integrated.

While collecting all previously provided data, including the tumor staging performed, a template-based textual finding is generated to save user time. All

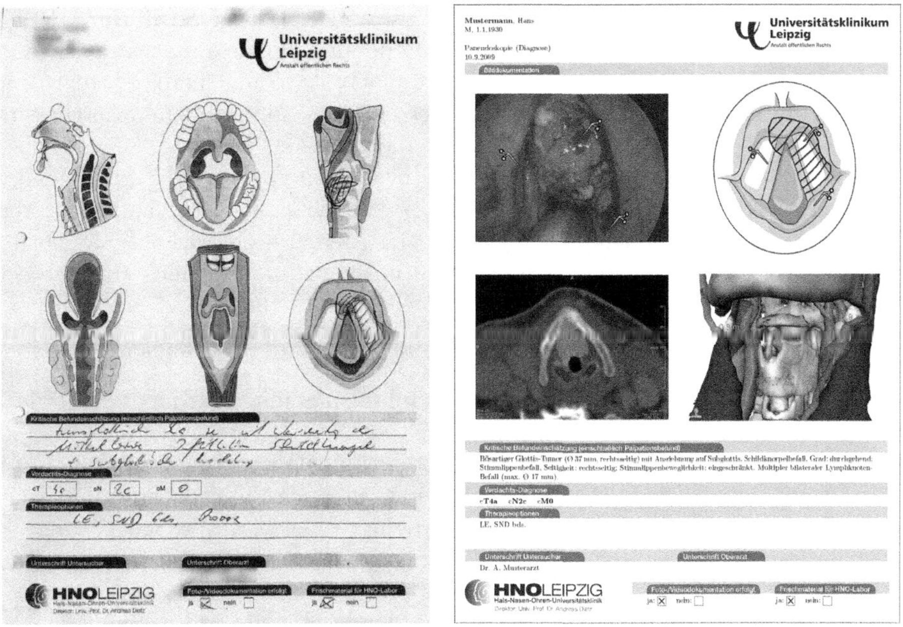

Fig. 7. *Left:* Handwritten report. Four of six schematic drawings stay completely unused. Moreover, the handwriting is barely readable. *Right:* Electronic report. Only the meaningful schematic drawings are included. Photos, relevant CT slices and dedicated scene views are directly integrated into the document. Though not printable, also an interactive 3D model can be embedded. Endoscopy photos and schemes are enriched with helpful annotations (like important regions, biopsy positions, tissue movability and further haptic findings). Finally, the electronic text is much better readable.

information can be altered and captured screenshots can be inherited and reordered prior to invoking report generation.

5 Clinical Use

The TTM was developed and refined with the help of our clinical partners. Their expertise relies on a falling number in ENT tumor surgeries – for 2009, an annual quantity of 280 tumor initial diagnoses was reported. Although a clinical study aiming at an in-depth workflow-analysis is still running, some interim results and trends can be provided already.

The TTM has been used by 8 surgeons, mainly at the ENT department in Leipzig, for planning more than 100 neck surgery interventions so far. In most cases, a selected set of functions was used to visualize and quantify the tumors in their spatial surrounding. In some 40 cases, the full set of functions (including virtual endoscopy and documentation) were used.

The computer-assisted planning process was mostly performed in addition to the conventional one based on CT and paper. This was primarily done to serve comparison of the different workflows, and the TTM is at times being used exclusively now. The computer-assisted planning process is accomplished in difficult cases where the tumor disease is at a later stage and therefore treatment is particularly challenging (two out of three patients exhibit a tumor in the late stages III and IV, and ten percent exhibit metastasis).

Only in rare cases (less than 5%) the overall surgical strategy was finally changed w. r. t. radicality or access. Yet, a significant rate of change for the clinical decisions when using vs. not using this software-tool was actually not to be expected, for this would have meant that until now the clinicians were subject to considerably wrong decisions on a more or less regular base. Nevertheless, the surgeon feels much safer with the computer-assisted planning and generally better prepared for surgery.

The TTM is considered particularly useful for planning treatment of surgical interventions at the larynx, because all relevant target structures (cricoid and thyroid cartilage) can be segmented and discriminated well in CT data. With respect to oropharynx, not all relevant structures can be separated and thus the 3D visualization is less helpful at present. This, however, may change if segmentation is instead (or additionally) based on other modalities like MRT or PET/CT.

The surgeons employing the system report an observable added-value w. r. t. multiple aspects. The use of a common DICOM viewer is mentioned to be a big advantage over needing to deal with all the different ones coming along with DICOM CDs. Measurements are reported highly vitally, but are used for 3D much more than for 2D slice view. Annotation functionalities, in turn, are in general considered very helpful. The biggest value is thereby added by the fast and easily annotatable endoscopy photos and schematic pictograms. Altogether, the surgeons appreciate the distinct but user-friendly documentation features allows for the first time to communicate precisely the results of examinations like the panendoscopy, in particular the estimated depth-infiltration of vascular structures and other tissue (recall Fig. 4). The involved surgeons report that with these functions they perform endoscopy more consciously and profoundly, since more findings can be reported.

It turned out that, discounting the effort for segmentation, the computer-assisted planning process is about 2min slower than the conventional one. This is in part due to the present need for manually entering patient information, importing CT data and endoscopy photos, etc. With a planned system-integration for PACS and HIS, additional time savings can be expected. Yet, since the expenditure of time stays within inter-surgery setup-times, the computer-assisted planning process fits into the clinical workflow. It has to be noted that the segmentation process, performed in advance, is quite time consuming at present (about 30min). Nevertheless, especially for difficult cases, the use of the TTM is already being preferred to the conventional planning and documentation, for it leads to findings of much higher expressiveness.

6 Conclusion

Treatment planning in case of severe diseases is a challenging process where many decisions have to be met with respect to the selected therapies, their combination and sequence. The required information can be derived from most different medical data modalities. Since all of these modalities have their individual advantages and disadvantages, a combination and exploitation of all available information is desired. The slice-based investigation of tomography data provides a raw insight into the leison and is familiar to virtually any clinician. 3D representations, in turn, approve better descriptions of small and complex structures (relation of cervical lymph nodes to vessels and skull base) and structure-based semantic interpretation of the image data (extent of malignant tissue, minimal distance to risk structures in neck surgery). Finally, the integration of additional non-radiological information (visual and palpatory findings and histological results) completes the surgeons mental model.

Providing means for collecting, combining and re-using information from different modalities, the TTM thus offers a real added value for ENT surgical planning and documentation. However, the reported gain in perceived safety is in fact highly subjective to the individual surgeons. A desirable profound quantification of the achieved or achievable improvements, in turn, is limited by the inherent problem that examinations like the panendoscopy are actually not repeatable in the real setting. Up to now, no details are known on precision or deviation of reporting tumor finding and therapy decision. To overcome this issue, a dedicated panendoscopy phantom [13] is currently in development that will offer a way for performing panendoscopy examinations under identical predefined conditions and measuring the deviation of examination results in the context of a known ground truth.

Despite the long-term effort described here, still not all clinical needs are fulfilled in an optimal way. In some hospitals, ultrasound or MRI are primarily used for diagnosis and treatment planning. Thus, it is desirable to adapt visual computing solutions to the peculiarities of such data. Advanced multimodal visualization, including information derived from different image data is at least in some hospitals a useful extension. In particular, if radiation treatment or chemotherapy are part of the overall treatment plan, treatment response has to be carefully evaluated which gives raise to comparative visualization solutions highlighting how the shape and size of tumors have changed over time.

Nevertheless, the described development process and the derived needs are likely a good basis for a variety of surgical and interventional procedures. In particular, an in-depth task analysis with a strong focus on the clinical workflow and with user stories as a major means to communicate the process and its variants turned can be considered instrumental and has proven successful also in the development of a surgical training system [14]. Yet, we do not overgeneralize our experiences. Each disease, diagnosis and treatment has in fact its very own certain peculiarities that need to be identified, interpreted and considered.

References

1. Dornheim, L., Dornheim, J., Rössling, I.: Complete Fully Automatic Model-based Segmentation of Normal and Pathological Lymph Nodes in CT Data. International Journal for Computer Assisted Radiology and Surgery 5(6), 565–581 (2010)
2. Dornheim, J., Lehmann, D., Dornheim, L., Preim, B., Strauß, G.: Reconstruction of Blood Vessels from Neck CT Datasets using Stable 3D Mass-Spring Models. In: Eurographics Workshop on Visual Computing for Biology and Medicine (EG VCBM), pp. 77–82 (2008)
3. Krüger, A., Tietjen, C., Hintze, J., Preim, B., Hertel, I., Strauß, G.: Interactive Visualization for Neck Dissection Planning. In: IEEE/Eurographics Symposium on Visualization (EuroVis), pp. 295–302 (2005)
4. Tietjen, C., Meyer, B., Schlechtweg, S., Preim, B., Hertel, I., Strauss, G.: Enhancing Slice-based Visuaizations of Medical Volume Data. In: IEEE/Eurographics Symposium on Visualization (EuroVis), pp. 123–130 (2006)
5. Tietjen, C., Preim, B., Hertel, I., Strauss, G.: A Software-Assistant for Pre-operative Planning and Visualization of Neck Dissections. In: Proceedings of CURAC, pp. 176–177 (2006)
6. Fischer, M., Strauß, G., Gahr, S., Richter, I., Müller, S., Burgert, O., et al.: Three-dimensional Visualization for Preoperative Planning and Evaluation in Head and Neck Surgery. Laryngorhinootologie 88(4), 229–233 (2009)
7. Boehm, A., Dornheim, J., Müller, S., Strauß, G., Wichmann, G., Dietz, A., et al.: TTM Tumor Therapy Manager. In: Proceedings of CURAC, Düsseldorf, pp. 17–20 (2010)
8. Carroll, J.M.: Making Use: Scenarios and Scenario-Based Design. In: Proceedings of the 3rd Conference on Designing Interactive Systems: Processes, Practices, Methods, and Techniques, DIS 2000, p. 4. ACM, New York (2000)
9. Rössling, I., Cyrus, C., Dornheim, L., Boehm, A., Preim, B.: Fast and Flexible Distance Measures for Treatment Planning. International Journal for Computer Assisted Radiology and Surgery 5(6), 633–646 (2010)
10. Rössling, I., Hahn, P., Cyrus, C., Dornheim, L.: Estimation of the Midsagittal Plane for Sideness Determination of Malignant Structures of Head and Neck. In: Eurographics Workshop on Visual Computing for Biology and Medicine (EG VCBM), pp. 109–115 (2010)
11. Edge, S.B., Byrd, D.R., Compton, C.C., Fritz, A.G., Greene, F.L., Trotti, A. (eds.): AJCC Cancer Staging Handbook: from the AJCC Cancer Staging Manual, 7th edn. Springer, Heidelberg (2009)
12. Sobin, L.H., Gospodarowicz, M.K., Wittekind, C.: UICC: TNM classification of malignant tumors, 7th edn. Wiley-Blackwell, Oxford (2009)
13. Boehm, A., Grunert, R., Möckel, M., Dietz, A., Zenou, E., Strauß, G.: Développent d'un fantôme pour la panendoscopie. Annales Françaises d'Oto-Rhino-Laryngologie et de pathologie cervico-faciale 127(4, suppl. 1), A30 (2010), 117e congrès de la SFORL, Paris, Octobre 16-18, 2010 - Hors-série
14. Cordes, J., Hintz, K., Franke, J., Bochwitz, C., Preim, B.: Conceptual Design and Prototyping Implementation of a Case-based Training System for Spine Surgery. In: Hambach, S., Martens, A., Urban, B. (eds.) Proc. of the 1st International eLBa Science Conference (e-Learning Baltics), Rostock, pp. 169–178 (2008)

An Image-Guided Surgery System to Aid Endovascular Treatment of Complex Aortic Aneurysms: Description and Initial Clinical Experience

Graeme Penney[1], Andreas Varnavas[1], Neville Dastur[2], and Tom Carrell[2,*]

[1] Department of Imaging Sciences and Biomedical Engineering, King's College London, St Thomas' Hospital, SE1 7EH, UK
{graeme.penney,andreas.varnavas}@kcl.ac.uk
[2] Department of Vascular Surgery, Guy's and St Thomas' NHS Foundation Trust, London, UK
neville@surgeons.org.uk, tom.carrell@gstt.nhs.uk

Abstract. We have designed an image guidance system to aid complex aortic aneurysm procedures. The system is based around an intensity-based 2D-3D rigid registration algorithm which accurately aligns a vertebra in the preoperative CT to interventional fluoroscopy. A 3D surface rendering of the aorta and relevant target vessels is then overlaid onto the fluoroscopy to aid guidance during the procedure. We report results from use of the system during twenty three procedures over a ten month period. Results showed the system to have an overall failure rate of 5.8%, which was mostly caused by errors in determining a starting position (misidentifying a vertebra). In 78% of cases our method was within our target accuracy of 3mm. Non-rigid deformation caused by the interventional instruments is believed to be the main reason for larger errors. In twenty one of the twenty three cases the surgeon rated the system as aiding the procedure.

1 Introduction

Endovascular stent-graft repair of aortic aneurysms was developed in the 1990s to provide a minimally-invasive alternative to open surgery, and in recent years has become a popular first-line treatment option. Endovascular grafts require a landing zone above and below the aneurysm to ensure an adequate seal and exclusion of the aortic bloodflow from the aneurysm sac, see figure 1(a). If the aneurysm lies close to, or crosses, the ostia of the visceral vessels (renal, superior mesenteric and celiac arteries), a standard endovascular graft cannot be used without compromising these important vessels. These anatomical restrictions have led some to conclude that a large proportion of patients are unable to benefit from endovascular treatment. Currently most patients with these

* Thanks go to the Guy's and St Thomas' charity for funding this work, and to our patients for participating in the study.

R.H. Taylor and G.-Z. Yang (Eds.): IPCAI 2011, LNCS 6689, pp. 13–24, 2011.

anatomically-challenging aneurysms are offered conventional open surgery, however recent advances in stent design have led to a new approach that offers a minimally-invasive option even in these complex cases. These "complex endovascular repairs" require the use of special, usually bespoke, stent-grafts which have openings (termed fenestrations, scallops or branches) for each of the visceral vessels involved, see figure 1(b). Accurate alignment of these complex endovascular grafts is essential to success as malpositioning is liable to occlude bloodflow to vital organs and carries a high risk of renal failure, intestinal ischaemia, liver failure and death. Covered 'bridging' stents are used to secure the main stent-graft to each of the vessel ostia in order to securely fix the alignment, thereby ensuring both preservation of flow to the target vessels and exclusion of the bloodflow from the aneurysm. These complex endovascular repairs require a higher level of precision than standard repairs, where the consequences of minor maldeployment are usually less serious.

Accurate alignment and deployment involves multiple procedural steps and is performed under x-ray guidance using iodinated contrast to enhance the target vessels while fine adjustments are made. The guidance may be further complicated because the initial positioning of the part-deployed stent-graft often

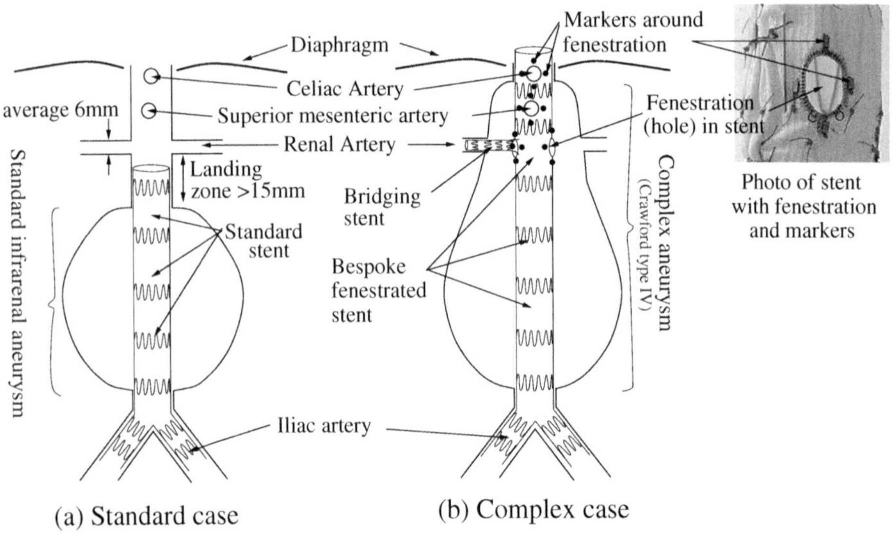

Fig. 1. Overview of standard (a) and complex (b) endovascular treatment of aortic aneurysms. Standard treatment (a) requires a landing zone (distance between top of aneurysm and renal arteries) of at least 15mm. The stent-graft consists of a fabric covered wire mesh, which is placed to exclude the aneurysm from the aortic bloodflow. Complex cases (b) occur when the aneurysm extends across the renal, superior mesenteric and/or celiac arteries. These cases require a bespoke stent-graft designed with fenestrations for each vessel. Once the main stent graft is deployed bridging stents (only one shown) are used to link the main stent with each artery, to secure stent-graft position and to isolate the aneurysm from aortic bloodflow.

inadvertently covers vessel ostia, preventing contrast-enhancement and visualisation of the target vessels.

The clinical imperative of accuracy combined with the difficulties in visualising target vessels led us to hypothesise that endovascular treatment of complex aortic aneurysms would benefit from additional information provided by an image-guided surgery (IGS) system. This paper describes the IGS system we have built, and reports on initial clinical experience of the system being used live during twenty three interventions.

Work carried out over ten years ago assessed the usefulness of an IGS system for *standard* endovascular repair of aortic aneurysms [1]. This concluded that a required accuracy of 1mm was needed, and this would be unachievable in 3D from a single view. We disagree with this previously proposed accuracy requirement, particularly for complex cases. We believe that accuracy of our system should be measured in terms of overlay accuracy i.e. a 2D projection accuracy, not a true 3D accuracy, as this is how information will be presented to the clinician. Fenestrated and branched endovascular aneurysm repair is a relatively novel clinical technique and we sought the opinion of specialists performing this procedure who considered that an error of half the diameter of the smallest common target vessel (renal artery 6mm, see Figure 1(a)) would be acceptable, and so set our target clinical accuracy to be 3mm.

Although there is a large amount of literature covering 2D-3D registration methods [6], there are far fewer publications describing 2D-3D image-guided surgery systems which have (or are) being used clinically. Exceptions are in radiotherapy, where commercial systems from Accuray (Cyberknife system) [4] and Brainlab (Novalis) now routinely use 2D-3D automatic intensity-based image registration to calculate patient position. Commercial systems are available to align preoperative CT to fluoroscopy images, via an intraoperative 3D rotational angiography image (i.e. a 3D-3D registration), which are in use for neuro applications [5], and such a system has very recently been reported for our target application: complex endovascular repair of aortic aneurysms [3]. Another area where 2D-3D image registration is making clinical impact is to aid navigation during cardiac electrophysiological procedures. Initial registration can be achieved either by precalibration, as in the case of the X-MR system [9], or by manual alignment (Philips EP navigator).

2 Materials and Methods

A prospective clinical study was set up in accordance with our national and institutional research ethics and governance procedures. A schematic overview of preoperative and intraoperative components of our IGS system is presented in Figure 2. Each of these components are now described in detail.

2.1 Preoperative CT Image Processing

Our registration algorithm matches on a single vertebra. To speed up computation regions of interest are defined in the CT scan around each vertebra relevant

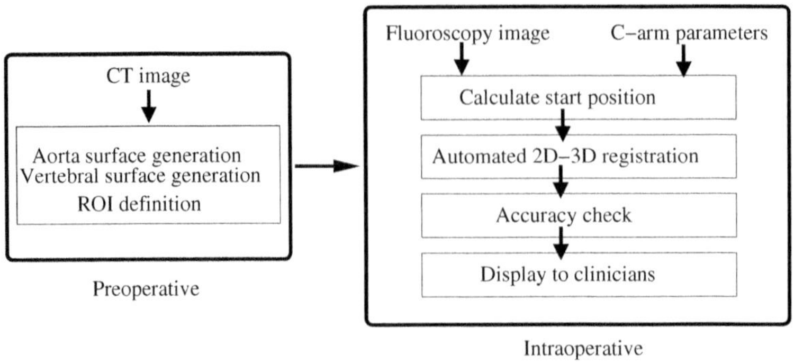

Fig. 2. Overview of IGS system. Preoperative stage (left) processes the CT image to define registration regions of interest (ROI), and creates surfaces for visualisation. Intraoperative stage (right) uses the preoperative stage output and the fluoroscopy image and C-arm position. The defined four processes are carried out in series to overlay the clinically relevant anatomy from CT onto fluoroscopy.

to the procedure. These are defined by extracting a rectangular region (size 80×80×40mm) around a point picked in the centre of each relevant vertebra.

In addition, a basic representation of each relevant vertebra, comprised of three orthogonal planes (see Figure 3), is manually produced using ITK-SNAP [10][1]. Relevant vertebrae are chosen depending upon aneurysm size and position. Vertebrae adjacent to the visceral vessels (L1/L2 and T12) are always involved. If the aneurysm extends to the aortic bifurcation L4 and L5 are included. Likewise if the aneurysm extends into the thorax then more thoracic vertebrae will be processed.

A surface of the aorta lumen and visceral vessels is produced from CT using the semi-automatic segmentation available in ITK-SNAP. Visceral vessels which will be preserved are segmented to beyond their first bifurcation. In cases where the patient has multiple vessels where only one will be preserved, the other vessels are only segmented a short distance. This is to help identify the situation where a guidewire has entered the wrong vessel.

2.2 Intraoperative Processing

Calculation of starting position. Images are acquired from a Siemens Axiom Artis DTA fluoroscopy system using a Sensoray 2255S USB frame grabber. At the moment of image capture four parameters are recorded from the fluoroscopy system, field of view (FOV), source-to-image distance (SID) and rotations of the C-arm (RAO/LAO right(left)-anterio-oblique angle and cranial-caudal (CC) angulation). From visual inspection a vertebra is identified on which to base the registration and this information is all input into a graphical user interface

[1] www.itksnap.org

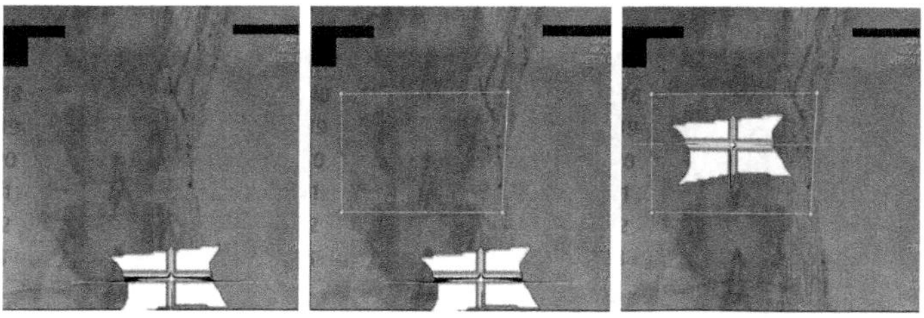

Fig. 3. Defining a start position. Initial position (left). Region of interest in 2D (yellow box) is drawn by picking four points in the fluoroscopy image which encompasses the chosen vertebra (centre). The chosen 3D CT vertebra surface is manually translated over the fluoroscopy vertebra (right) to complete the process.

(GUI) written in c++ with use of VTK[2]. Figure 3 describes the full process which takes approximately twenty seconds.

2D3D image registration. An intensity-based 2D3D registration algorithm is used. The algorithm produces synthetic 2D images from the CT known as digitally reconstructed radiographs (DRRs) which are compared with the fluoroscopy image using a gradient difference similarity measure [7]. The main difference between this algorithm and a previously published version [7] is a new optimisation strategy. To improve capture range and robustness an initial coarse global optimisation strategy is used (described in detail below). The best position from the global search is then taken and refined using a simple hill climbing search strategy.

The global optimisation splits the six registration parameters into three in-plane and three out-of-plane parameters, as described in figure 4. The out-of-plane parameters are altered by each combination of the following amounts: $\pm 5°$ and $\pm 10°$ for θ_x, θ_y and ± 100mm and ± 200mm for X, resulting in 125 positions and a DRR produced. Each of these DRRs are then taken and an in-plane registration is carried out between the DRR and fluoroscopy image. Again a global optimisation strategy is used, translating over half the size of the region of interest drawn around the vertebra (described in section 2.2) in ± 10 steps, and rotating $\pm 10°$ in steps of $2°$, resulting in 4851 positions per DRR. Overally, 606,375 similarity measure values are calculated during the global optimisation.

Accuracy check: Registration accuracy is checked by visual inspection of vertebra features between the fluoroscopy image, and an overlaid DRR produced at the registration position.

Display to clinicians: Our computer's video card output is connected to one of the three monitors directly in front of the clinicians during the procedure. Our display allows the clinician to request: the surface overlay to be faded in and out;

[2] www.vtk.org

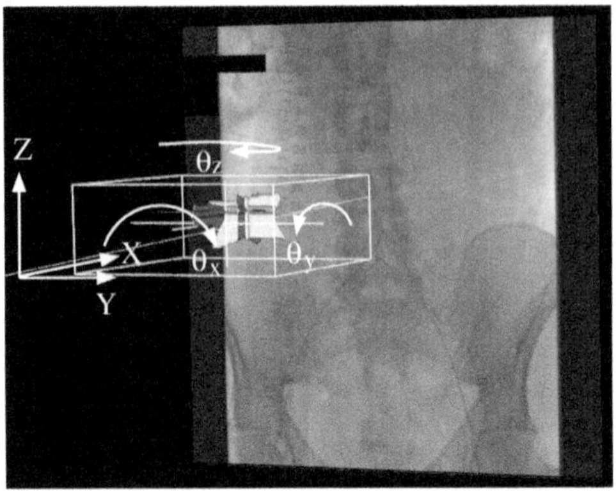

Fig. 4. CT position and orientation is defined by six rigid body parameters, three translations X, Y, Z, and three rotations $\theta_x, \theta_y, \theta_z$. These can be split into parameters which define movements parallel to the plane of the fluoroscopy image (in-plane parameters θ_x, Y, Z) and parameters which define movements a component of which is normal to the fluoroscopy plane (out-of-plane parameters θ_y, θ_z, X).

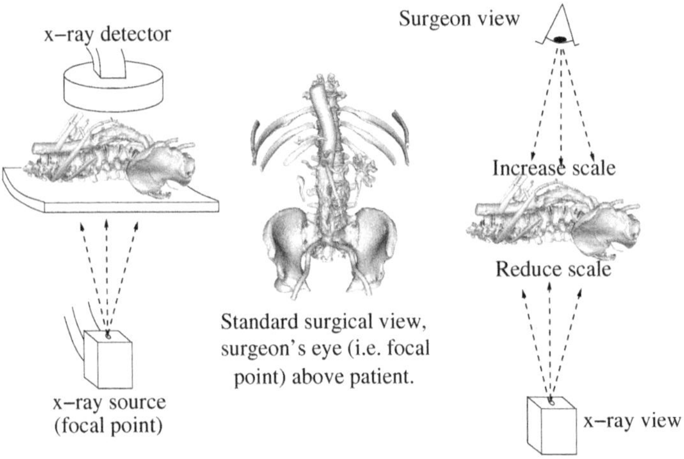

Fig. 5. Reverse-perspective procedure. X-ray images are typically acquired with the x-ray source below the patient (left), however the standard surgical view is from above the patient (centre). This is achieved by flipping the fluoroscopy image about its vertical axis. To go from the geometrically correct x-ray view to the surgical view it is necessary to carry out a variable scaling process perpendicular to the source-to-film direction where features close to the x-ray source are reduced in size, while features further from the x-ray source are enlarged. This is followed by two reflections, a flip about the fluoroscopy vertical axis and a flip along the x-ray source to film direction.

points picked on the surface to be projected onto the fluoroscopy; points picked on the fluoroscopy to be presented as a line back-projected through the surface; and the surface to be rotated to provide some 3D information. We display the aorta from the standard clinical viewpoint (from above the patient), whereas, the x-ray source (i.e. the pin-hole in our perspective projection model) is usually situated below the patient. To achieve the correct mapping between 3D and 2D from the clinical viewpoint it is necessary to carry out a "reverse-perspective" procedure which entails deforming the 3D surface as detailed in figure 5.

2.3 Experimental Method

Our system has been run live during twenty three complex endovascular aortic repairs over a ten month period. On average fifteen registrations were carried per procedure at approximately regular intervals or when specifically requested by the surgeon. Mean registration time was 169 sec on a single 3MHz CPU. The vast majority of the registrations were to low-dose screening fluoroscopy images. Information on aorta deformation due to interventional instruments was obtained by visual comparison of the overlay and a digital subtraction angiography image.

3 Results

Robustness results are summarised in Table 1. The majority of failed registrations were due to user error, in particular 11 failures (55% of total failures) were due to misidentifying the vertebra. Locating the correct vertebra is particularly difficult in the thorax and from lateral views. Eight of these failures occurred in a single case where the patient had an anatomical variation which confused the operator (patient had an extra lumbar vertebrae and a large spur rib on L1) resulting in no successful registration for that case. Once the anatomical variation was pointed out, the system performed accurately. From the other failures three were due to incorrectly positioning the vertebra, and six were failures in the automated registration algorithm which are discussed in figure 6. Failed registration images were not used in the subsequent accuracy analysis below. The much higher failure rate ($8 \times$ larger) using just simple hill-climbing optimisation clearly shows the benefit of our initial global optimisation method.

Table 1. Summary of algorithm robustness broken down into manual user error (predominantly misidentiifying a vertebra) and algorithm failures. Algorithm failures are reported for our new algorithm with the inital global optimisation detailed in section 2.2, and for comparison, using the old hill-climbing optimisation [7].

Number of Registrations	Number of failures due to:		
	User error	Algorithm failure	
		New global optimisation	Old hill-climbing optimisation
344	14 (4.1%)	6 (1.8%)	52 (15.7%)

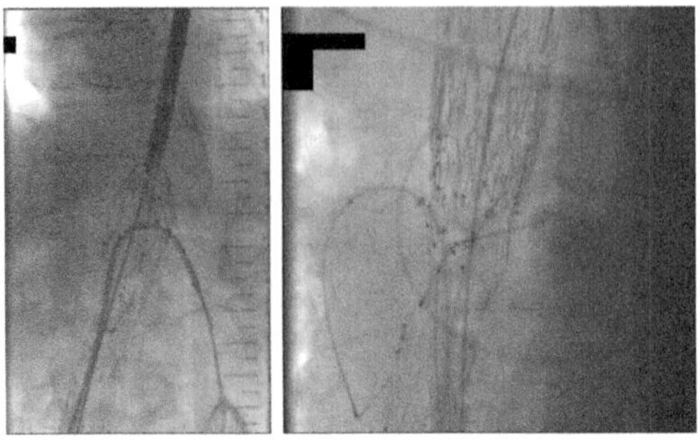

Fig. 6. Example images for which registration failed. Three failures occurred for AP views (an example is shown above left). Three failures occurred from lateral views (example shown above right), probably due to lack of features from spinous processes (which greatly aid registration).

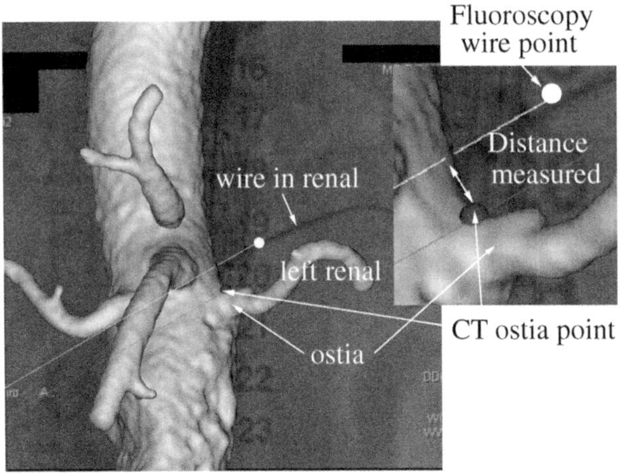

Fig. 7. Demonstration of accuracy calculation. If ostia did not directly overlay the wire then the point closest to the wire was picked on the ostia (red dot) and projected onto the fluoroscopy (red line). The closest wire point to this projection was picked (white dot) and projected back into 3D (white line). Error distance measured was the minimum distance between the red dot and white line (know as reprojection distance).

Overlay accuracy was measured on a subset (between 1 and 4) of images from each patient dataset which clearly showed a guidewire within a specific vessel. Accuracy was calculated by comparing the position of overlay vessel ostia with the fluoroscopy position of the guidewire. Zero error was recorded if the wire went through the ostia overlay. Otherwise, the minimum distance the ostia needed to be moved to overlay the wire was calculated as described in Figure 7.

Accuracy results were calculated for the starting position and final registration position, see Figure 8. The registration algorithm can be seen to have greatly increased the percentage of cases which showed zero error and reduced the number of high error cases. The mean accuracy was 1.7mm for the final position, and 78% of cases had errors of 3mm or less. Three example fluoroscopy images and overlays are presented in Figure 9.

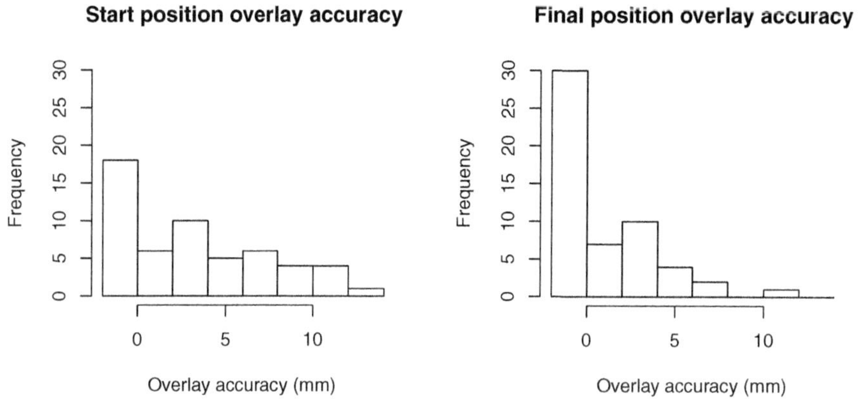

Fig. 8. Histograms of overlay accuracy measured at vessel ostia. Zero values denote wire from fluoroscopy was inside CT overlay of ostia. Values above zero show minimum movement required to place wire inside ostia. Results on left show starting position accuracy. Results on right show final accuracy after 2D3D image registration.

4 Discussion

Our initial hypothesis was that endovascular treatment of complex aortic aneurysms could be aided by an image-guided surgery system. We have presented results from our 2D-3D image guidance system over a series of twenty three patients who underwent complex aortic aneurysm procedures. Although the study has been performed on a single site, subjective feedback from the operating surgeon and radiologists during these cases supports our hypothesis. In all except two cases (one where the system failed to register and one where the vessels were all easy to find) the clinicians stated that the system aided the procedure. The specific benefits cited by the clinicians were:

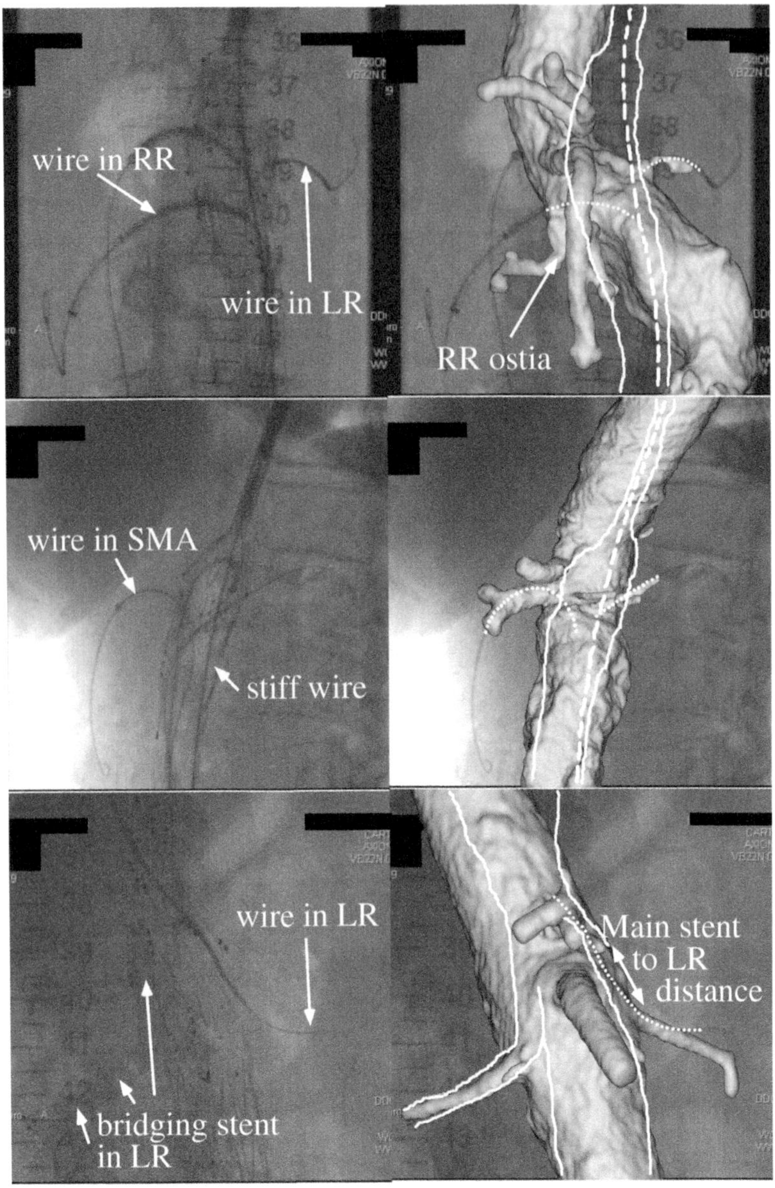

Fig. 9. Example fluoroscopy (left) and corresponding overlay images (right). To improve clarity the following features have been highlighted in overlay images: wires in vessels (white dotted lines); stiff wire within aorta (dashed white line); edges of stent-graft (solid white lines). Top pair of images show largest error in 23 patient series. The right renal (RR) ostia is 12mm from the wire. Note the local nature of the deformation as the left renal (LR) wire is accurately aligned. Middle pair show accurate alignment for superior mesenteric artery (SMA) and left renal. Bottom pair show accurate alignment for both renals in a branched case. One of the uses of the system is due to the long distance between the main stent and the artery in branched cases.

– Guiding endovascular graft position and orientation to optimise graft and target vessel alignment in order to aid cannulation.
– Selecting landing zones for bridging stents in target vessels.
– Confirming cannulation of the correct renal artery in cases with multiple renal arteries.
– Identifying wire malposition in the false lumen of one patient with chronic aortic dissection.

Our system is currently operated by experienced researchers. For the system to be used more widely (i.e. at different sites) and for direct control by clinicians, we believe work is required in the following three areas:

1. An improved method to determine a starting position. Our current method requires identification of specific vertebra. One solution would be to initially register on a wide field-of-view fluoroscopy, where vertebrae would be easy to identify, and then use a separate tracking system, (e.g. Philips EP navigator) to maintain registration (or provide starting positions) for different views.
2. To speed up the registration. This is currently being tackled by implementation of the software on graphics processing units.
3. Identification of failed registrations. Our current method using visual inspection, which has worked well for our purposes, but would probably be inadequate for less experienced users.

The accuracy difference between histograms in Figure 8 shows the benefit of using automated registration, compared to basic manual positioning. Our manual starting position assumes patients lie in the same position on the fluoroscopy and CT tables. Registration results showed that patient rotations of 3-4° occurred on average (max 8°) between CT and fluoroscopy positions.

The main contribution to overlay error is non-rigid motion caused by the stiff wires and device delivery systems lying inside the aorta. A preliminary pilot study, involving retrospective 2D-3D registration (eleven patients), showed a strong correlation between overlay error and aorta angulation [2]. Preliminary work applying a manually picked landmark thin-plate-spline deformation to the aorta showed that it was possible to reduce errors to below 5mm even for highly angulated aortas [8]. We aim to investigate more sophisticated methods for non-rigid registration, in particular the application of a finite element model to warp the aorta to overlay the position of interventional instruments within the aorta.

5 Conclusion

Image guidance can aid complex endovascular repair of aortic aneurysms. Early results using our 2D-3D registration algorithm has demonstrated accuracy and robustness during twenty three fenestrated and branched endovascular aneurysm repairs. Clinician feedback has described significant subjective benefit in helping to achieve procedural success and, on their request, we will continue to use and develop this system during these complex procedures. Further work is needed to simplify identification of a starting position, to accelerate the algorithm and to incorporate a reliable automated method of identifying false registrations.

References

1. Breeuwer, M., Wadley, J.P., de Bliek, H.L.T., Desmedt, P.A.C., Gerritsen, F.A., Gieles, P., Buurman, J., Dorward, N.L., Velani, B., Kitchen, N.D., Thomas, D.G.T., Wink, O., Blankensteijn, J.D., Eikelboom, B.C., Mali, W.P.T.M., Viergever, M.A., Penney, G.P., Gaston, R., Maurer, Jr., C.R., Hill, D.L.G., Hawkes, D.J., Maes, F., Vandermeulen, D., Verbeeck, R., Suetens, P., Weese, J., Sabczynski, J., Zylka, W., Lorenz, C., Buzug, T.M., Schmitz, G., Kuhn, M.H.: The EASI Project—Improving the effectiveness and quality of image-guided surgery. IEEE Trans. Inform. Technol. Biomedicine 2, 156–168 (1998)
2. Carrell, T., Modarai, B., Brown, J., Penney, G.: Feasibility and limitations of an automated 2D-3D rigid image registration system for complex endovascular aortic procedures. J. Endovasc. Ther. 17, 527–533 (2010)
3. Dijkstra, M., Eagleton, M., Greenberg, R., Mastracci, T., Hernandez, A.: Intra-operative C-arm cone-beam computed tomography in fenestrated/branched aortic endografting: A preliminary experience. J. Vasc. Surg. (2010); article in press, Epub. ahead of print available
4. Fu, D., Kuduvalli, G.: A fast, accurate, and automatic 2D-3D image registration for image-guided cranial radiosurgery. Med. Phys. 35(5), 2180–2194 (2008)
5. Lin, C., Blanc, R., Clarençon, F., Piotin, M., Spelle, L., Guillermic, J., Moret, J.: Overlying fluoroscopy and preacquired CT angiography for road-mapping in cerebral angiography. Am. J. of Neuroradiology 31, 494–495 (2010)
6. Markelj, P., Tomaževič, D., Likar, B., Pernuš, F.: A review of 3D/2D registration methods for image-guided interventions. Med. Image Anal. (2010) (in press)
7. Penney, G.P., Weese, J., Little, J.A., Desmedt, P., Hill, D.L.G., Hawkes, D.J.: A comparison of similarity measures for use in 2D-3D medical image registration. IEEE Trans. Med. Imaging 17(4), 586–595 (1998)
8. Raheem, A., Carrell, T., Modarai, B., Penney, G.: Non-rigid 2D-3D image registration for use in endovascular repair of abdominal aortic aneurysms. In: Medical Image Understanding and Analysis, pp. 153–157 (2010)
9. Rhode, K., Hill, D., Edwards, P., Hipwell, J., Rueckert, D., Sanchez-Ortiz, G., Hegde, S., Rahunathan, V., Razavi, R.: Registration and tracking to integrate x-ray and MR images in an XMR facility. IEEE Trans. Med. Imaging 22(11), 1369–1378 (2003)
10. Yushkevich, P.A., Piven, J., Cody Hazlett, H., Gimpel Smith, R., Ho, S., Gee, J.C., Gerig, G.: User-guided 3D active contour segmentation of anatomical structures: Significantly improved efficiency and reliability. Neuroimage 31(3), 1116–1128 (2006)

OR Specific Domain Model for Usability Evaluations of Intra-operative Systems

Ali Bigdelou, Tobias Sterner, Stefan Wiesner, Thomas Wendler, Florian Matthes, and Nassir Navab

Technische Universität München

Abstract. Studying the usability of a system has become increasingly popular over the last decades and is seen as a crucial factor for the success of many systems and products. In a complex domain, like the Operating Room, creating systems with high usability is even more important, as deficiencies in the design can have serious impacts. However, evaluating the usability of systems in complex domains like the Operating Room (OR) is not an easy endeavor. In order to handle the complexity of the OR domain, usability specialists require deep domain knowledge, which they usually cannot acquire.

To support the usability study of intra-operative systems, we propose an OR specific domain model and inspect how this model could be used to reduce some of the usability evaluation problems. The proposed model consists of various aspects of the Operating Room, which affect the domain complexity like workflow, human role and their interconnections. As a proof of concept, we report from a usability study of an intra-operative device, which was performed based on the proposed approach.

1 Introduction

Usability study is becoming more and more popular during recent years and in many cases it is even turning to an official governmental constraint for the industries [1,2]. It has been shown that reducing usability problems has a direct impact on the overall functionality of a system [1,3]. The usability factor in medical domains such as Operating Room plays a more critical role due to the fact that any mistake can lead to a serious problem. Because of the contribution of novel technologies to the modern healthcare systems, medical staff has to deal with an increasing number of complicated medical devices, which raises the risk of errors, possibly leading to adverse events, i.e. injuries caused to patients as the result of a medical intervention rather than the underlying medical condition. According to an estimation published by an Institute of Medicine report, between 44,000 to 98,000 people die each year from preventable medical errors in American hospitals [4]. These figures exceed the annual number of fatalities caused by motor vehicle accidents, breast cancer, or AIDS. Although a lot of these errors are not related to medical devices, some are directly or indirectly linked to their use. Other studies, have shown that 69% of the adverse events are rooted in wrong usage of technical equipment [5].

R.H. Taylor and G.-Z. Yang (Eds.): IPCAI 2011, LNCS 6689, pp. 25–35, 2011.

Since deficiencies in the design of medical technology can increase the risk of human error [6], healthcare systems need to be designed carefully. For frontline clinicians, who make life-affecting decisions every day, medical devices are only valuable if they make their job easier. Systems which increase their workload or the chance of error will not be tolerated [7]. Consequently, designers strive for devices with high usability standards, by applying systematic usability engineering techniques [3,8].

Several definitions of usability have been presented [1,3,9], all consisting of a set of components. Nielsen describes usability using the components *learnability*, *efficiency*, *memorability*, *errors*, and *satisfaction* [3]. The aim of usability studies is to improve the *user interface* of a system in regards to the *usability components* of interest. A variety of methodologies to evaluate the usability of a system's user interface have been proposed. In [10], Ivory et al. propose *testing*, *inspection*, *inquiry*, *analytical modeling* and *simulation* as five main classes of *usability evaluation* methods. *Testing* methods are regarded as the most fundamental way to evaluate usability [3]. They refer to all *evaluation methods*, which involve *test users* working with the target system within a controlled environment. Test subjects perform predefined tasks with a fully developed product or a prototype, while being observed by evaluators. There are numerous methods to conduct a usability test such as *thinking-aloud*, *performance measurements*, and *log file analysis* [10,11]. The idea behind the *thinking-aloud* method is that test subjects continuously verbalize their thoughts, while interacting with the system. This results in a considerable amount of qualitative data.

There are some studies about *usability evaluation* in medical environments. Liljegren has investigated the importance of the Nielsen's usability components in medical context [12]. Based on his work, the most significant component for the medical staff is the *errors* factor. Moreover he proposed *usability tests* as the most appropriate *evaluation method* for medical devices since they fulfill all relevant criteria and are also able to cover all components of usability. In [8], Kushniruk et al. describe the *usability testing* methodology they have applied and refined over the past ten years for the evaluation of health information systems, such as a computer-based patient record system (CPR).

Despite the fact that usability engineering techniques are successfully applied in many domains, creating systems with high usability can be a tremendous challenge in *complex domains* like the OR [13]. Chilana et al. argues that workers in *complex domains* require deep subject-matter knowledge and experts insights [14]. Their work consists of open ended and unstructured problems [13], and comprises many unique situations. When studying the usability of a system, it is crucial to have a complete understanding of the domain the system is used in. Yet in *complex domains*, this is not a simple endeavor [14].

Complex domains impose challenges during all steps of conducting a usability test. Within the *planning* phase, usability experts report difficulties in knowing where and how to begin, asking the right questions, developing realistic tasks, and understanding new domain-specific concepts [14]. While *executing* the test, usability specialists struggle to interpret the relevance and significance of observed problems. Furthermore, compared to non-complex domains, the *analysis* and *reporting* process require additional time and effort.

Considering the potential impact, which the usability of healthcare devices entails in regards to patient outcomes and the challenges posed to usability engineers when evaluating medical systems, the need for an approach to support their work becomes clear. In this work we aim at introducing an OR specific domain model which could be incorporated into a usability study of intra-operative systems. By combining the proposed model with a usability engineering process, we try to overcome some of the challenges faced by usability engineers in the OR domain and alleviate the process of performing usability evaluations of intra-operative devices. We will evaluate the proposed approach during a usability study of an intra-operative imaging device.

2 Modeling Approach

In this section we introduce the proposed OR domain model to overcome some of the mentioned challenges of usability studies in the OR. It has been shown that the complexity of a domain may be rooted, among other things, in the interaction of multiple users and system components, and the presence of unforeseen events [13]. We propose to tackle this complexity by decomposing the OR domain into the main aspects responsible for complexity and by establishing a clear connection between the defined fragments. The generated domain can later be used to facilitate usability studies in the OR.

Our conceptual representation of the OR domain consists of several key components. The first component is a *view*, which is used to capture a single source of complexity in the OR domain. Next for each proposed *view* of the OR, we also introduce a proper *representation*. Then, based on these *view representations*, we define corresponding *view elements*. These elements embody aspects relevant to usability engineers, when focusing on the respective *view*.

To create a proper domain model, we first carefully study the OR in close collaboration with domain experts, i.e. surgeons and technical experts of the field, e.g. providers of intra-operative devices. After analyzing the state of art in the modeling of the OR [15,16,17,6], we identified three key components (*views*) of the OR domain, which can be considered as the primary sources of complexity for usability evaluations. These are *workflow*, *human role* and the *intra-operative device* itself.

The *workflow* of an intervention encompasses the common steps of one type of surgery, determining the tasks of each involved role and the use of surgical devices. A *surgical workflow* may be captured manually during field observations and interviews with surgeons or with automatic OR workflow recovery methods [18,6]. When developing an intra-operative device, it is crucial to consider that the system has to integrate smoothly into the current *workflow* of an intervention and support surgical activities. If a system does not adapt to the surgical routine, it may not be accepted by the surgeons. Furthermore, *surgical workflow* is affected by the characteristics of a device and may be altered in case a system introduces new treatment opportunities. For these reasons, we see *workflow* as one of the key aspects of intra-operative usability evaluations, and therefore include it as a *view* in our model of the OR domain. In order to represent this *view*, we model the *workflow* as a simple flow chart, describing the distinct steps of a surgery, as depicted in figure 1.a. Moreover, we define the workflow stages as *view elements* within this *view* of the model.

Many advanced surgical devices can be used simultaneously by multiple users with different *roles*. Depending on the *human role*, different tasks may be performed with the system. As the background of each *human role* can vary, diverse types of information or different ways of visualization may be required. Obviously, this introduces a high degree of complexity for usability studies, which is why we consider *human roles* as the second *view* in our model. Each entity is a distinct *human role*, which has to be included as an element within the *human roles view*. The entities have to be defined according to the *human roles*, which are actually involved in a particular type of surgery, e.g. surgeon, nurse, anesthetist and circulator.

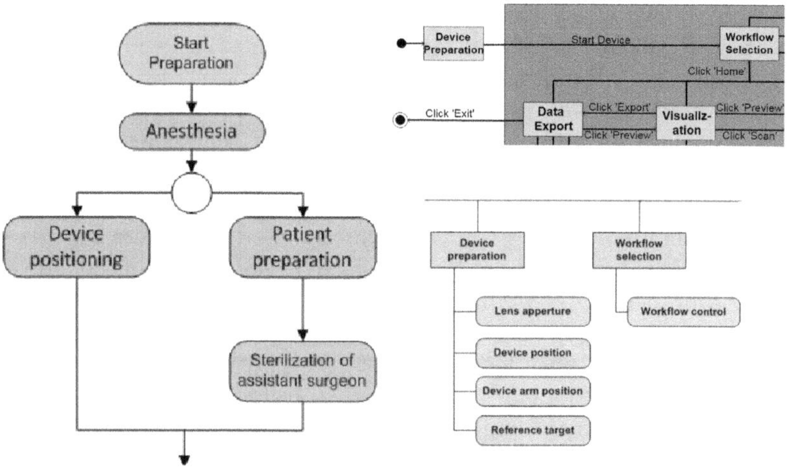

(a) (b)

Fig. 1. (a) An examplary surgical workflow flow chart, (b) top, a state machine diagram; bottom, a feature tree diagram, describing device states and related features.

Due to recent technological advances, intra-operative devices have turned into complex systems. They provide a number of advanced functionalities, facilitating surgical procedures. As the functions of such devices are tightly coupled with the current *workflow stage* and the *human roles* interacting with the system, the third *view* in our domain model covers the *target device* itself. We describe a surgical device by two entities, *features* and *states*. A *feature* is defined as a functionality or part of the system, which should be investigated during an evaluation. Depending on the objectives of the study, the granularity degree of *features* can vary from low level user interface elements (e.g. record button, cancel button, and progress bar), to high level abstractions, which summarize several components (e.g. record controls). *Features* are encompassed in logical units called *states*. For modeling the *states* of a device we use a state machine diagram, as illustrated in figure 1.b-top. To represent the available *features* for each *state*, we used a simple feature tree as can be seen in figure 1.b-bottom. An element in the *device view* consists of a pair *device feature* and corresponding *device state*.

To model the interconnections between various *views*, we further define *mapping* in our model. A *mapping* is defined as the correlation between two *elements* of different *views*. The relationship of the *elements* can be specified through attributes, which may be derived from the view context. The set of possible *mappings* between the *elements* of two *views* are encapsulated within a *mapping table*. As these tables abstract the complex connections between views, they provide the opportunity to easily map *elements* of one *view* to another, and hence allow usability engineers to evaluate and observe the domain, based on various perspectives. Figure 2.a illustrates how the *views* and the *mapping tables* are integrated into our model of the OR domain.

3 Integration in the Usability Engineering Process

The amounts of *test data* gathered during a usability evaluation can be enormous. In this work, by *test data* we refer to any data produced during the whole process of a usability evaluation like *test tasks*, *evaluation objectives*, and *comments of users* about the device usability. In every domain, the findings of a usability test are highly dependent on the expertise of the evaluator, especially during *data analysis*. As this data only contains low level facts and figures, careful interpretation is necessary to extract useful information. In complex domains, analyzing *test data* is an even bigger challenge, as the complexity of the domain is embodied in the gathered data. As usability professionals do not possess thorough domain knowledge, it is hard for them to perceive the potential correlations between the *test data* and the domain.

In order to tackle this problem, we propose to incorporate any data involved during a usability test into the OR domain model. This can be accomplished by binding *test data* elements to the *elements* of a *view*, as can be seen in figure 2.b. Since the *mapping tables* of our model allow for a transition between existing *views*, it is sufficient to connect the test data to only one *view*. The most effective way to do this is using the *device view*, as the *data elements* will usually relate to a certain *features* of the device. This helps to identify potential correlations between the observed data and the domain. Therefore, the task of retrieving meaningful information from the *test data* is simplified.

During the *planning* phase, once the evaluation objectives have been defined, they should be integrated into the OR model. Each objective can be bound to relevant *elements* of the available *views*. This allows for an observation of the objectives in the context of the model. Furthermore, this information can assist in the arrangement of the study design.

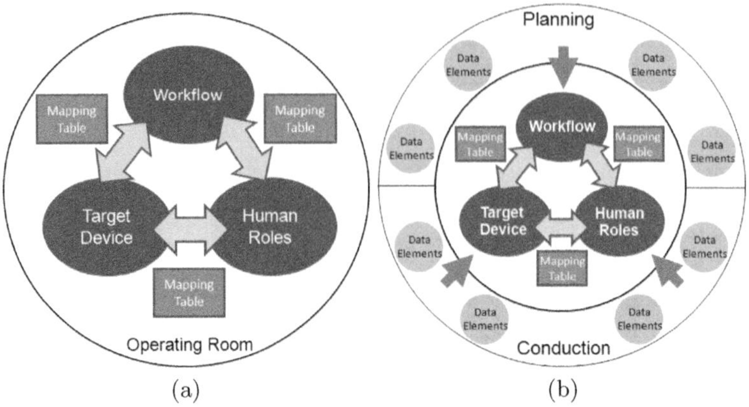

Fig. 2. (a) The proposed OR domain model for usability study, (b) an instance of the domain model with incorporated *test data* gathered within the *planning* and *conduction* phases of a usability test

In order to acquire significant information, it is important to define appropriate *tasks* within a meaningful context for test subjects. The identified *test tasks* represent data, which should be integrated into the model, as it may allow usability specialists to see how these tasks cover different aspects of the domain. In the course of usability *tests sessions*, subjects are commonly given a subset of possible *test tasks*. As the set of *test tasks* has been mapped to our model, the conductor is able to see how the current tests cover *elements* of any *view*. In case not all areas of the domain are covered sufficiently, he may alter the tests accordingly.

For the *analysis* of the collected comments, evaluators need to handle a vast range of data. Retrieving appropriate information is a challenging task, especially in a complex domain. By applying our modeling approach, the basis for a comprehensive analysis is set. In combination with an appropriate visualization technique, our model can facilitate the test data analysis. Since the findings from the evaluation have been connected to the model, the evaluator can easily navigate through the collected data, connect them in a meaningful way, and interpret the information in the context of the available views. As an example, the evaluator can see the impact of the identified problems on different stages of the *workflow* or on specific *human roles*.

4 Experiments: Case Study

In this section we report on the usability study of an intra-operative imaging device, which was performed using our proposed model. We conducted a usability test on an intra-operative SPECT imaging device in context of the Sentinel Lymph Node Biopsy (SLNB). This procedure is relevant in a variety of clinical cases, including breast cancer and melanoma. The SPECT imaging device is used to create a 3D SPECT image directly in the OR. The system also superimposes this information on live video images within the OR. This visualization allows the surgeon to find and dissect the SLNs.

We instantiated our model by capturing 23 *workflow stages* of the SLNB [19,20,21], identifying 5 involved key *human roles* and 45 *device features*, grouped in 8 *device states*. After modeling the three *views* for the given context, the *mapping tables* have been produced accordingly. The study has been performed in close collaboration with our industrial partners and cooperating surgeons of our university hospital.

The test was conducted with 7 participants, who have been selected with various level of domain expertise. Figure 3.a illustrates the layout of the test environment. A patient phantom (P) was placed on a table (4) in the center of the test room, covered by surgical sheets. Two cameras (1, 2) were used to record the test scenery and the screen of the imaging device. The device (3) was placed next to the head of the phantom. The test conductor (C) was seated behind the dummy patient, instructing and observing the session. Figure 3.b shows a photo of the test environment.

Each test was conducted as a standard usability test session [11], lasting between 30-40 minutes, involving a formal greeting, an introduction and a signing of agreements. Each subject was asked to perform a subset of 15 defined *test tasks*, while all interactions were recorded. During this procedure, the conductor did not interfere or answer questions, unless the subject could not continue the assigned task independently.

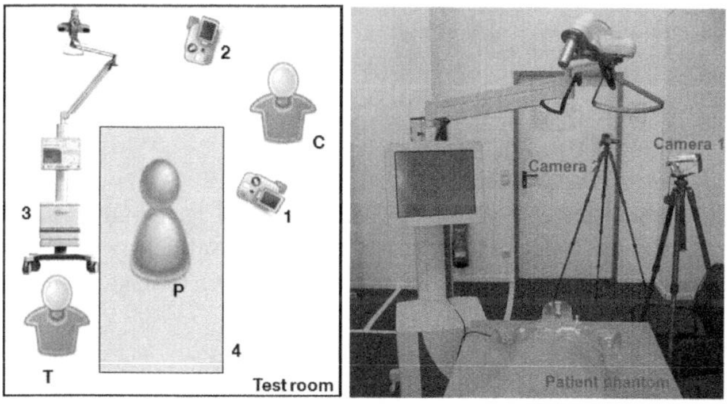

(a) (b)

Fig. 3. (a) Layout of the test environment, (b) a picture showing the test lab

After completing the test sessions, all the comments made by users about usability of the device were collected. Furthermore we categorized them as *complaints*, *suggestions*, *positive feedbacks*, *help requests*, *general comments*, *bugs* and *observations*. In total, 94 individual comments have been made. Each comment item has been bound to the corresponding device feature. Due to the mappings between the three OR model views, each item can be analyzed in the context of affected workflow stages and the human roles. This enabled us to study all comments related to a workflow stage particularly important for the overall success of the surgical intervention. Moreover, during each workflow stage, we were able to find out about the challenging aspects of the device from the perspecitve of every individual role. As an example, a comparatively high number of complaints has been made regarding the device preparation stage. Further investigation revealed the circulator as the mainly affected role. This highlighted device features which require further improvement.

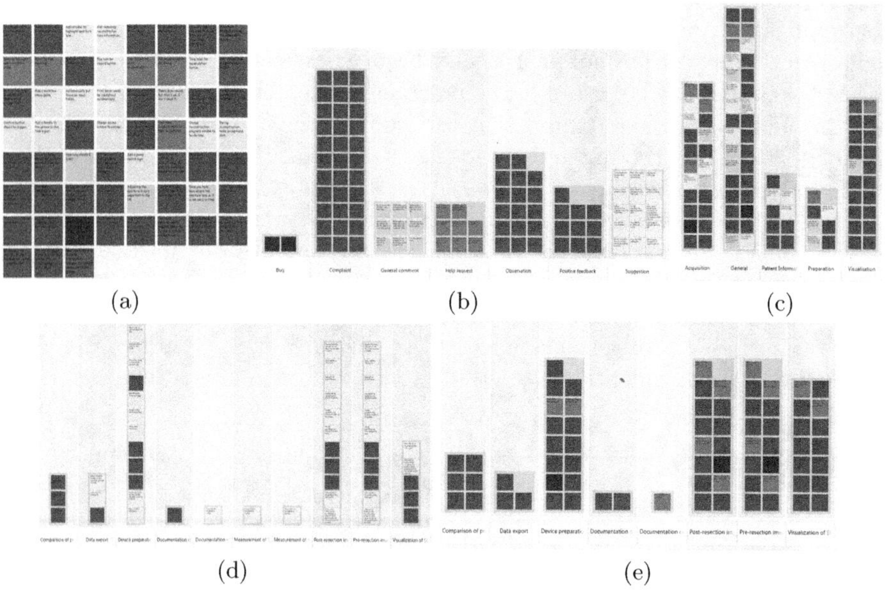

Fig. 4. Examplary screenshots of Pivot, showing (a) all gathered usability comments, (b) comments sorted by type, (c) the distribution of comments over *workflow stages*, (d) positive comments / suggestions over *workflow stages*,(e) negative comments / help requests / bugs over *workflow stages*

Having the collected data bound to the defined OR model, it is possible to benefit from these structured data in different ways. One option is to use a proper data visualization technique to make it possible for usability engineers to find problems and weaknesses of the system as well as their impact to the overall procedure. Another approach could be to develop an automatic processing algorithm, which identifies and prioritizes all the problems in the system based on their overall impact.

In this work we took the first approach, and utilized a recently developed visualization methodology called PivotView [22]. 4.a shows a subset of comments made by users in Pivotview. Each comment is represented by one colored item containing it's essential message. The color indicates the comment type. By combining our model with the visualization power of PivotView, these items can be organized based on the comment types as shown in figure 4.b. The mapping tables of our model enable us to visualize the feedback based on various parameters defined in the model. For example, 4.c is representing the distribution of comments over workflow stages. Moreover, the filtering feature of PivotView allowed us to selectively study the positive and negative comments, as can be seen in figure 4.d-e. During the interpretation phase, this structured visualization of comments helped us to identify usability problems of the target system.

5 Discussion

As mentioned before, the *usability data* gathered during different phases of the usability study could be mapped into the proposed model. Having such a structured data with its underlying domain model, usability engineers can analyze and evaluate usability problems in the context of the OR domain. In this part we outline some of the main benefits of this approach.

1. *Communication Base:* A structured domain specific model of the OR would make it possible for industrial engineers, who might not be familiar with advanced medical terminology, to easily identify main aspects of the domain. As many of the specific medical terms, like those used for specifying *workflow stages*, could be retrieved from the model, it could be used as a non-formal basis for communication, facilitating the interaction with medical staff.

2. *Test task definition:* Furthermore the model could be used during the creation of *test cases*, to investigate whether *test tasks* properly cover the different *workflow stages* of the procedure and to select tasks, which are representative for the involved *human roles*.

3. *Conduction:* Based on the results of preceding test sessions, our modeling approach helps to pick test tasks for the next participant, coresponding to those *device features*, *workflow stages*, and *human roles*, which had not yet been covered sufficiently.

4. *Analysis and interpretation:* The *analysis* and *interpretation* steps were highly simplified, as the model *views* allowed us to investigate the collected data in the context of the OR domain, revealing the potential impact of identified problems. Using the structured model behind the usability data, it is possible to see how comments of the users are distributed among various *workflow stages*, or how many help requests any of the involved *human role* has. Furthermore, by filtering irrelevant data the usability engineers can have a closer look on other aspects of the domain, which are affected by the currently examinded *device feature.*

5. *Less dependency to domain experts:* Once the proposed model is completed in close collaboration with experts, it does capture the domain knowledge. Therefore, the need for continuous consulting of specialists is partially eliminated. This also results in a reduction of the dependency on the evaluator's particular domain knowledge.

The reader is encouraged to study the complementary video material for getting further insight into the proposed model.

6 Conclusion

In this work we proposed a context specific domain model for usability study in the Operating Room. The proposed model contains detailed information about the target system and its environment, which can be incorporated during many steps of a usability test. It introduces the three main views for OR as *surgical workflow*, *human role* and *target device*. This method shows promising results of considering the OR domain model during the production of intra-operative devices. Further investigation could be done on automating different steps of the proposed method.

References

1. ISO IEC 62366. Medical devices – Application of usability engineering to medical devices (2007)
2. Hodgson, P.: Usability for medical devices: A new international standard, Available online at `http://www.blueprintusability.com/topics/articleiec62366.html` (visited on October 4, 2010)
3. Nielsen, J.: Usability Engineering. Morgan Kaufmann Publishers, San Francisco (1994)
4. Wachter, R.M.: The end of the beginning: Patient safety five years after 'to err is human'. Health Affairs (2004)
5. Backhaus, C.: Usability-Engineering in der Medizintechnik: Grundlagen - Methoden - Beispiele. Springer, Heidelberg (2010)
6. Blum, T., Padoy, N., Feußner, H., Navab, N.: Workflow mining for visualization and analysis of surgeries, Barcelona, Spain, pp. 134–135 (June 2008)
7. Wiklund, M., Wilcox, S.: Designing Usability Into Medical Products. CRC, Boca Raton (2004)
8. Kushniruk, A.W., Patel, V.L.: Cognitive and usability eng. methods for the evaluation of clinical info. system. J. of Biomedical Informatics 37(1), 56–76 (2004)
9. Seffah, A., Donyaee, M., Kline, R.B., Padda, H.: Usability measurement and metrics: A consolidated model. Software Quality Journal 14(2), 159–178 (2006)
10. Ivory, M.Y., Hearst, M.A.: The state of the art in automating usability evaluation of user interfaces. ACM Computing Surveys 33, 470–516 (2001)
11. Kjeldskov, J., Skov, M., Stage, J.: A longitudinal study of usability in health care: Does time heal. Int. J. of Medical Informatics 79(6), e135–e143 (2010)
12. Liljegren, E.: Usability in a medical technology context assessment of methods for usability evaluation of medical equipment. International Journal of Industrial Ergonomics 36(4), 345–352 (2006)
13. Redish, J.: Expanding usability testing to evaluate complex systems (2006)
14. Chilana, P.K., Wobbrock, J.O., Ko, A.J.: Understanding usability practices in complex domains. In: CHI 2010: Proceedings of the 28th International Conference on Human Factors in Computing Systems, pp. 2337–2346. ACM, New York (2010)

15. Ohnuma, K., Masamune, K., Yoshimitsu, K., Sadahiro, T., Vain, J., Fukui, Y., Miyawaki, F.: Timed-automata-based model for laparoscopic surgery and intra-operative motion recognition of a surgeon as the interface connecting the signal scenario. Int. J. Com. Assist. Radiol. Surg. 1(1), 442–445 (2006)
16. Bouarfa, L., Stassen, L., Jonker, P., Dankelman, J.: Discovery of surgical high-level activities in the operating. In: ASCI 2010 (2010)
17. Neumuth, T., Strauß, G., Meixensberger, J., Lemke, H., Burgert, O.: Acquisition of process descriptions from surgical interventions. In: Database and Expert Systems Applications, pp. 602–611 (2006)
18. Rosen, J., Brown, J., Chang, L., Sinanan, M., Hannaford, B.: Generalized approach for modeling minimally invasive surgery as a stochastic process using a discrete markov model. IEEE Trans. on Biomedical Eng. 53(3), 399–410 (2006)
19. Santi, I., Fantini, L., Herrmann, K., Fuccio, C., Wendler, T., Caroli, P., Castelucci, P., Buck, A.K., Schwaiger, M., Fanti, S.: Freehand spect for sentinel lymph node biopsy: clinical experience. In: EANM 2010, Vienna, Austria. EANM (October 2010)
20. Wender, T.V.: 3d intraoperative functional imaging with navigated probes (2010)
21. Buck, A.K., Ehlerding, A., Saeckl, J., Herrmann, K., Wendler, T., Martignoni, M.E., Schnelzer, A., Schwaiger, M.: Evaluation of feasibility of freehand spect in the or. In: Proceedings of the EANM 2010, Vienna, Austria. EANM (October 2010)
22. Microsoft Live Labs Pivot: Pivot Viewer (2010), `http://www.microsoft.com/silverlight/pivotviewer/`

A Multi-view Active Contour Method for Bone Cement Reconstruction from C-Arm X-Ray Images

Blake C. Lucas[1,2], Yoshito Otake[1], Mehran Armand[2], and Russell H. Taylor[1]

[1] Dept. of Computer Science, Johns Hopkins University
Baltimore, Maryland
[2] Johns Hopkins Applied Physics Laboratory
Laurel, Maryland
blake@cs.jhu.edu, {otake,rht}@jhu.edu,
mehran.armand@jhuapl.edu

Abstract. A novel algorithm is presented to segment and reconstruct injected bone cement from a sparse set of X-Ray images acquired at arbitrary poses. The Sparse X-Ray Multi-view Active Contour (SxMAC – pronounced "smack") can (1) reconstruct objects for which the background partially occludes the object in X-Ray images, (2) use X-Ray images acquired on a non-circular trajectory, and (3) incorporate prior CT information. The algorithm's inputs are pre-processed X-Ray images, their associated pose information, and prior CT, if available. The algorithm initiates automated reconstruction using visual hull computation from a sparse number of x-ray images. It then improves the accuracy of the reconstruction by optimizing a geodesic active contour. A cadaver experiment demonstrates SxMAC's ability to reconstruct high contrast bone cement that has been injected into a femur and achieve sub-millimeter accuracy with 4 images.

Keywords: Segmentation, Reconstruction, Active Contour, Deformable Models, Bone Cement, Intra-operative Imaging.

1 Introduction

The problem of recovering 3D shape from a sparse set of 2D projection images is common in interventional imaging. If prior information such as a statistical shape model is available, then this information may be used to assist in reconstruction [1]. However, such information is not always available, especially if the object is highly deformable or its shape is created and/or substantially modified during the procedure. Examples include surgical procedures for injecting cement into bones, such as vertebroplasty [2], sacroplasty [3], and femoroplasty [4].

Our immediate, focusing clinical application is femoroplasty, in which cement is injected into the neck and intertrochanteric area of the femur for patients with severe osteoporosis. The goal is to strengthen the femur to prevent fractures [4]. In our system (see Fig. 1) [5], preoperative CT images are used for preoperative planning, based on a 3D finite element analysis of the patient's femur and planned cement injection [6]. The preoperative model and plan are registered to the patient and

R.H. Taylor and G.-Z. Yang (Eds.): IPCAI 2011, LNCS 6689, pp. 36–46, 2011.

intraoperative navigation system using 2D-3D registration from intraoperative x-rays, and a robotic device is used to inject cement containing an appropriate contrast agent. At various stages during the injection, a sparse set of intraoperative x-rays (at most 8, but preferably 4) are taken of the cement and the cement volume in the bone is estimated. This information is used to repeat the finite-element analysis of augmented bone strength and to support re-planning and optimization for further injections. Conventionally, the shape of the cement volume is estimated by intersecting cones formed from the silhouettes of the cement in the images. However, the resulting models do not accurately reflect the actual cement volumes (e.g., Fig 4b). Our goal in this work is to significantly improve the accuracy of this reconstruction while still using only a small number of intraoperative x-rays from a conventional C-arm.

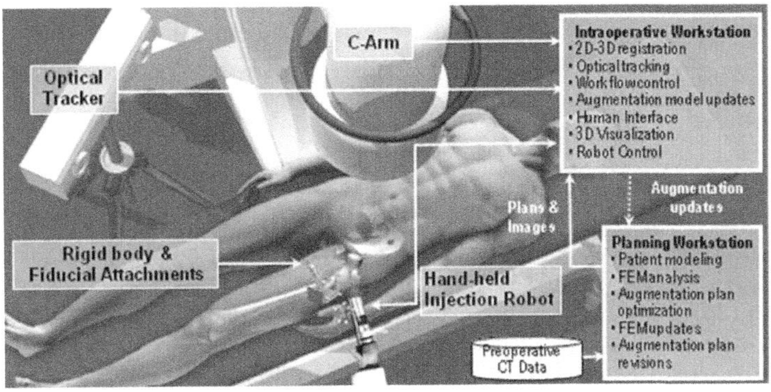

Fig. 1. System overview

2 Background

Techniques have been developed in computer vision to reconstruct objects observed from multiple viewpoints without prior information. One classical approach is to segment an object's silhouette in images, back-project the silhouettes into 3D space, and compute the intersecting volume. This technique is known as silhouette reconstruction or visual hull computation, and has been used in computer vision [7] and C-Arm X-Ray reconstruction [8]. It has been shown that the visual hull encloses all other reconstructions that can be explained by 2D segmentations of an object [9]. However, the visual hull may not and is unlikely to be consistent with observed image intensities of the object. The visual hull can be used to initialize more sophisticated approaches that generate reconstructions more consistent with image intensities. In particular, Geodesic Active Contours [10] reconstruct objects by optimizing an objective function on the image intensities that considers all observations of an object simultaneously [11, 12].

Active contour techniques have been extended to tomographic reconstruction [13] and CBCT [14-16]. In these methods, the segmentation process is formulated as the minimization of an objective function that incorporates information from acquired X-Ray images $\{I_k(\boldsymbol{x}_k) | \boldsymbol{x}_k \in D[k] \subset \mathbb{R}^2\}$ in log space, linear attenuation coefficients

$\{\mu(\boldsymbol{X})|\boldsymbol{X} \in D \subset \mathbb{R}^3\}$ in patient coordinates, and geometric properties of the deformable model:

$$E = E_{model}(\boldsymbol{X}) + E_{data}\big(\mu(\boldsymbol{X}), I_1(\boldsymbol{x}_1), \cdots, I_K(\boldsymbol{x}_K)\big). \tag{1}$$

In this paper, we formulate the segmentation process as an optimization problem that permits the segmentation algorithm to (1) reconstruct deformable objects for which the background partially occludes the object in X-Ray images, (2) use X-Ray images acquired on a non-circular trajectory, and (3) incorporate prior CT information. Subsequently, we describe a method for optimizing the objective function and evaluate the feasibility and performance of the Sparse X-Ray Multi-view Active Contour algorithm (SxMAC - pronounced "smack") to reconstruct injected bone cement. In particular, we're interested in knowing how many X-Ray images and how much contrast is required to achieve acceptable accuracy.

3 Method

3.1 SxMAC Algorithm

We formulate the reconstruction task as a global optimization problem that minimizes the following objective function, which describes the disparity between X-Ray images and Digitally Reconstructed Radiographs (DRRs) of a deformable model:

$$\begin{aligned} E_{data} = &\sum_{k}^{K} \int_{D[k]} \big(I_k(\boldsymbol{x}_k) - DRR_k\{\mu\}(\boldsymbol{x}_k)\big)^2 \mathrm{d}\boldsymbol{x}_k \\ &+ \int_D \lambda_{fg} |\nabla \mu_{fg}(\boldsymbol{X})|^2 \mathrm{H}_{fg}(\boldsymbol{X}) \\ &+ \lambda_{bg} |\nabla \mu_{bg}(\boldsymbol{X})|^2 \mathrm{H}_{bg}(\boldsymbol{X}) \mathrm{d}\boldsymbol{X} \end{aligned} \tag{2}$$

where,

$$DRR_k\{\mu\}(\boldsymbol{x}_k) = \int_D \mu(\boldsymbol{X})\, \delta\big(\boldsymbol{x}_k - \wp_k(\boldsymbol{X})\big) d\boldsymbol{X} \tag{3}$$

and,

$$\mu(\boldsymbol{X}) = \mu_{fg}(\boldsymbol{X})\mathrm{H}_{fg}(\boldsymbol{X}) + \mu_{bg}(\boldsymbol{X})\mathrm{H}_{bg}(\boldsymbol{X}) \tag{4}$$

and,

$$\mathrm{H}_{fg}(\boldsymbol{X}) = \Big(1 - \mathrm{H}\big(\omega_{bg}(\boldsymbol{X})\big)\Big)\Big(1 - \mathrm{H}\big(\omega_{fg}(\boldsymbol{X})\big)\Big) \tag{5}$$

and,

$$\mathrm{H}_{bg}(\boldsymbol{X}) = \Big(1 - \mathrm{H}\big(\omega_{bg}(\boldsymbol{X})\big)\Big)\mathrm{H}\big(\omega_{fg}(\boldsymbol{X})\big). \tag{6}$$

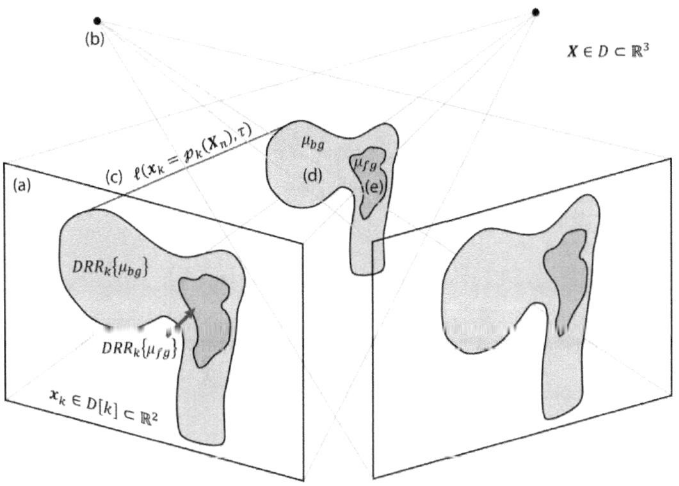

Fig. 2. Imaging scenario depicting (a) X-Ray images, (b) X-Ray source, (c) projection lines, (d) background objects, and (e) foreground object

Table 1. Definition of terms and expressions

Terms and Expressions	Definition
$\boldsymbol{x}_k \in D[k] \subset \mathbb{R}^2$	Pixel coordinates in the domain of image k.
$\boldsymbol{X} \in D \subset \mathbb{R}^3$	Patient coordinates in 3D.
$\boldsymbol{X}_n \in \mathbb{R}^3$	Position of the nth voxel in an image.
$\mathbb{I}_n \in \mathbb{R}^{1xN}$	Indicator vector for which the nth column is 1 and all other columns are 0.
$D_{fg}[k]$ and $D_{bg}[k]$	Foreground (fg) and background (bg) domains in X-Ray image k.
$\mu_{fg}(\cdot)$ and $\mu_{bg}(\cdot)$	Linear attenuation coefficients for foreground and background regions in 3D.
$I_k(\cdot)$	The log x-ray intensity image.
$H(\cdot)$	Heaviside function.
$DRR_k\{\mu\}(\boldsymbol{x})$	Simulated X-Ray image k generated from volume μ.
$vec(\boldsymbol{M})$	A column vector representing the elements of matrix $\boldsymbol{M}$.
$\delta(x) = \frac{d}{dx}H(x)$	Dirac delta corresponding to the Heaviside function $H(\cdot)$.
$\mathscr{p}_k(\boldsymbol{X})$	Mapping from patient coordinate space to pixel coordinates in image k.
$\boldsymbol{M}_k \in \mathbb{R}^{MxN}$	System matrix approximating the x-ray imaging equation.
$\omega_{fg}(\boldsymbol{X})$ and $\omega_{bg}(\boldsymbol{X})$	3D Level set corresponding to the foreground (fg) and background (bg) object. Level sets are negative inside the object and positive outside.
$\mathrm{H}_{fg}(\boldsymbol{X})$ and $\mathrm{H}_{bg}(\boldsymbol{X})$	Volumes indicating the foreground and background regions.
c_{fg} and c_{bg}	Constants describing foreground (fg) and background (bg) intensities.

The objective function E_{data} measures the L2 norm of the difference between simulated X-Ray images (μ) and the log of each x-ray image, subject to an L2 penalty on the smoothness of μ. The complete objective function, including data and geometric terms, is as follows,

$$E = \sum_{k}^{K} \int_{D[k]} \left(I_k(\boldsymbol{x}_k) - DRR_k\{\mu\}(\boldsymbol{x}_k)\right)^2 \mathrm{d}\boldsymbol{x}_k + \int_{D} \lambda_{fg} \left|\nabla \mu_{fg}(\boldsymbol{X})\right|^2 \mathrm{H}_{fg}(\boldsymbol{X}) + \lambda_{bg} \left|\nabla \mu_{bg}(\boldsymbol{X})\right|^2 \mathrm{H}_{bg}(\boldsymbol{X}) + \lambda_{\kappa} \delta\left(\omega_{fg}(\boldsymbol{X})\right) \left|\nabla \omega_{fg}(\boldsymbol{X})\right| \mathrm{d}\mathbf{X} \tag{7}$$

$DRR_k(\cdot)$ can be discretized and expressed as a weighted linear combination of $\mu(\boldsymbol{X})$:

$$DRR_k\{\mu\}(\boldsymbol{x}_k) = \sum_{\{\boldsymbol{X} | \boldsymbol{x}_k = \wp_k(\boldsymbol{X})\}} w_k(\boldsymbol{X}) \mu(\boldsymbol{X}) \tag{8}$$

or alternatively,

$$vec(DRR_k\{\mu\}) = \boldsymbol{M}_k vec(\mu). \tag{9}$$

$\boldsymbol{M}$ is an MxN matrix where M is the number of pixels in the X-Ray image and N is the number of voxels in μ. The matrix is completely defined by X-ray geometry (extrinsic and intrinsic parameters) and does not depend on the image or volume intensities. To efficiently solve eq. 7, let the foreground and background appearances be modeled as a constant (i.e. $\mu_{fg}(\boldsymbol{X}) = c_{fg}$ and $\mu_{bg}(\boldsymbol{X}) = c_{bg}$). The objective function simplifies to,

$$E = \sum_{k}^{K} \left\| vec(I_k) - c_{fg} \boldsymbol{M}_k vec\left(\mathrm{H}_{fg}\right) - c_{bg} \boldsymbol{M}_k vec\left(\mathrm{H}_{bg}\right) \right\|^2 + \int_{D} \lambda_{\kappa} \delta\left(\omega_{fg}(\boldsymbol{X})\right) \left|\nabla \omega_{fg}(\boldsymbol{X})\right| \mathrm{d}\mathbf{X} \tag{10}$$

The SxMAC model can be augmented to incorporate prior CT information by replacing the background indicator $\mathrm{H}_{bg}(\boldsymbol{X})$, with the prior CT ($\mu_{CT}$) :

$$\widetilde{\mathrm{H}}_{bg}(\boldsymbol{X}) = \mathrm{H}_{bg}(\boldsymbol{X}) \mu_{CT}(\boldsymbol{X}). \tag{11}$$

This extension assumes μ_{CT} is properly registered and intensity calibrated so that the background DRR is highly correlated with the background observed in acquired X-Ray images. $\mathrm{H}_{bg}(\boldsymbol{X})$ is a segmentation mask of the field of view that is common to both the prior CT and C-Arm acquisition that encloses the foreground $\mathrm{H}_{fg}(\boldsymbol{X})$. Solving the Euler-Lagrange equation for c_{fg} and c_{bg},

$$0 = \left.\frac{\partial E}{\partial c_{fg}}\right|_{c_{fg}} = -2\sum_{k}^{K} vec^{\mathrm{T}}(\mathrm{H}_{fg})\boldsymbol{M}_k{}^{\mathrm{T}}\left(vec(I_k) - \boldsymbol{M}_k vec(\mu)\right) \tag{12}$$

$\boldsymbol{M}_k$ and $\boldsymbol{M}_k{}^{\mathrm{T}}$ are referred to as forward and backward projection operators respectively. From eq. 12 we obtain,

$$\hat{c}_{fg}(c_{bg}) = \sum_{k}^{K} \frac{\left(\boldsymbol{M}_k vec(\mathrm{H}_{fg})\right)^{\mathrm{T}}\left(vec(I_k) - c_{bg}\boldsymbol{M}_k \mathrm{H}_{bg}\right)}{\left\|\boldsymbol{M}_k vec(\mathrm{H}_{fg})\right\|^2} \tag{13}$$

and similarly,

$$\hat{c}_{bg}(c_{fg}) = \sum_{k}^{K} \frac{\left(\boldsymbol{M}_k vec(\mathrm{H}_{bg})\right)^{\mathrm{T}}\left(vec(I_k) - c_{fg}\boldsymbol{M}_k(\mathrm{H}_{fg})\right)}{\left\|\boldsymbol{M}_k vec(\mathrm{H}_{bg})\right\|^2}. \tag{14}$$

The model's appearance can be optimized by alternating between $c_{fg} = \hat{c}_{fg}(c_{bg})$ and $c_{bg} = \hat{c}_{bg}(c_{fg})$ until convergence. Evolution of the deformable model's level set $\omega_{fg}(\boldsymbol{X})$ is computed by gradient descent [10],

$$\omega_{fg}^{t+1}(\boldsymbol{X}) = \omega_{fg}^{t}(\boldsymbol{X}) - \gamma \frac{\partial E}{\partial \omega_{fg}^{t}} \tag{15}$$

where,

$$\left.\frac{\partial E}{\partial \omega_{fg}}\right|_{\boldsymbol{X}=\boldsymbol{X}_n} = 2(c_{fg} - c_{bg})\delta\left(\omega_{fg}(\boldsymbol{X}_n)\right)\textstyle\sum_k^K \mathbb{I}_n \boldsymbol{M}_k{}^{\mathrm{T}}\left(vec(I_k) - \right. \tag{16}$$

$$\left.\boldsymbol{M}_k vec(\mu)\right) + \lambda_\kappa \delta\left(\omega_{fg}(\boldsymbol{X}_n)\right)\nabla\cdot\frac{\nabla\omega_{fg}(\boldsymbol{X}_n)}{|\nabla\omega_{fg}(\boldsymbol{X}_n)|}.$$

In the actual implementation, we do not store $\boldsymbol{M}_k$ and $\boldsymbol{M}_k{}^{\mathrm{T}}$ because they are very large sparse matrices. Instead, the graphics card is used to compute elements of those matrices on-the-fly using OpenCL.

3.2 Experiment Setup

We conducted a cadaver study to evaluate a surgical procedure in which bone cement is injected into an osteoporotic femur [5]. One objective of the procedure is to provide feedback to the surgeon via intra-operative reconstruction of the injected bone cement. Predictions about the post-operative structural properties of the femur can be made from its 3D reconstruction and pre-operative CT [6]. To this end, Pre and post operative CBCTs were acquired with a flat panel C-Arm. Geometric calibration followed the method described by Daly, Siewerdsen et al. [17].

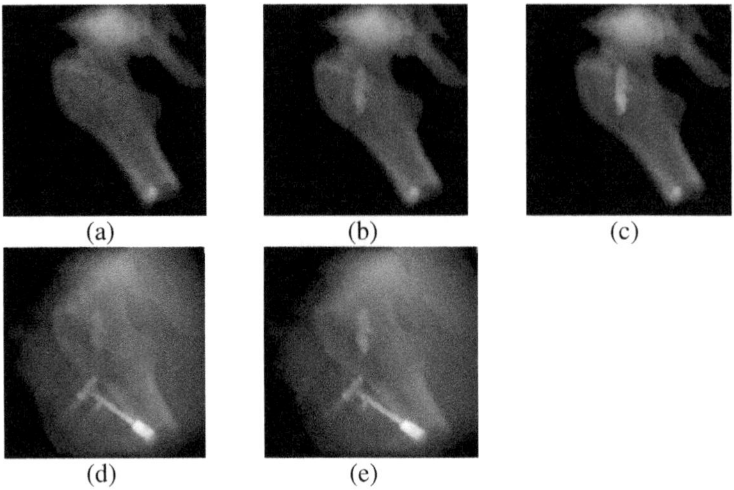

Fig. 3. (a) Synthesized pre-operative and post-operative X-Ray images with a cement attenuation of (b) 1730 HU without soft tissue; (c) 1900 HU without soft tissue; (d) 1730 HU with soft tissue; (e) 1900 HU with soft tissue

To evaluate the performance of SxMAC for this application, pre and post operative CBCTs were pre-processed to synthesize X-Ray images (Fig. 3).

Pre-processing was necessary to circumvent issues not addressed by SxMAC: 2D/3D registration of pre-operative CT to intra-operative X-Ray images and intensity matching between DRRs and acquired X-Ray images. CBCTs would not be acquired in a real clinical scenario; instead, a pre-operative diagnostic CT would be used as a prior. The following pre-processing steps synthesize pre and post operative CBCT and X-Ray images that are perfectly registered and intensity matched:

1. Pre-operative CBCT was registered to post-operative CBCT using intensity-based 3D/3D registration.
2. The femur was segmented in pre-operative CBCT.
3. The cement was segmented in post-operative CBCT and the Volume of Interest (VOI) was copied and pasted into the registered pre-operative CBCT.
4. DRRs for the CBCTs with and without the bone cement were generated.

4 Results

Experiments were conducted to evaluate SxMAC. In all cases, the deformable model was initialized by silhouette reconstruction with 8 images and bone cement attenuation[1] of 1900 HU. The initialization had a maximum error of 10 mm, and mean

[1] Attenuation measurements are approximate and do not correspond exactly to CT numbers because the CBCT from the C-Arm was not calibrated for this experiment. The peak cortical bone attenuation was measured at 1620 HU, and bone cement was measured at 1550 HU.

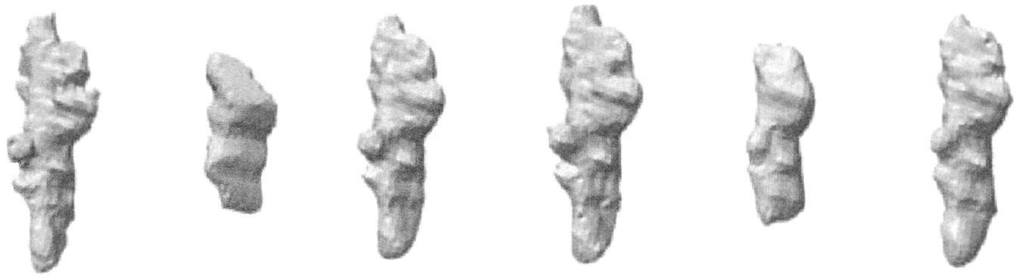

(a) (b) (c) (d) (e) (f)

Fig. 4. (a) Ground truth segmentation and (b) silhouette reconstruction. SxMAC reconstruction with 4 images and cement attenuation of (c) 1730 HU without soft tissue; (d) 1900 HU without soft tissue; (e) 1730 HU with soft tissue; (f) 1900 HU with soft tissue.

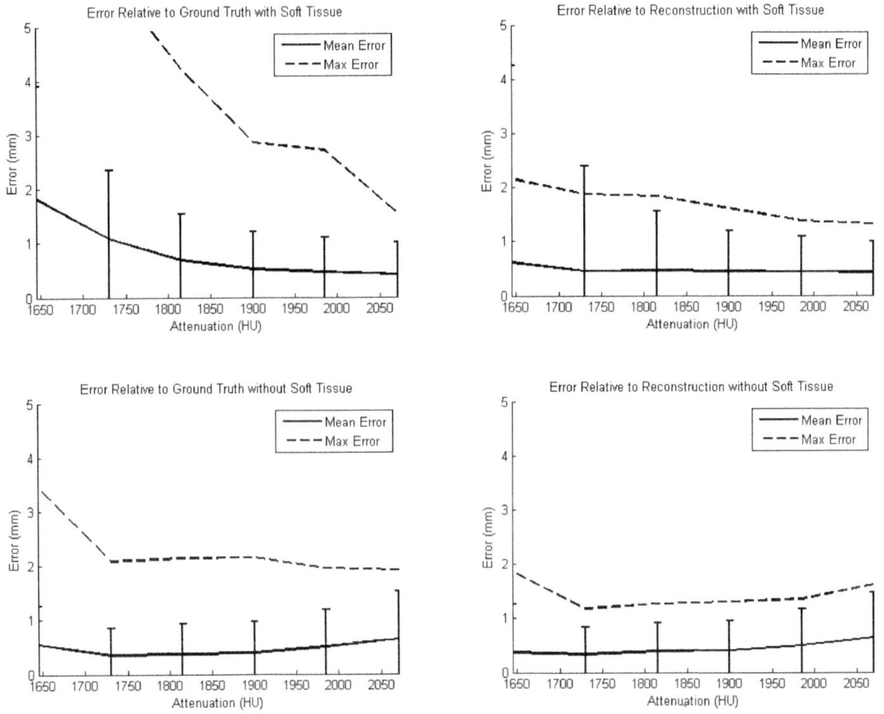

Fig. 5. Error between ground truth and SxMAC reconstruction for varying bone cement attenuation. The maximum error for silhouette reconstruction was 10 mm. The mean error was 2 mm and 0.77 mm for reconstruction-to-truth and truth-to-reconstruction measurements respectively. Error bars indicate one standard deviation from the mean.

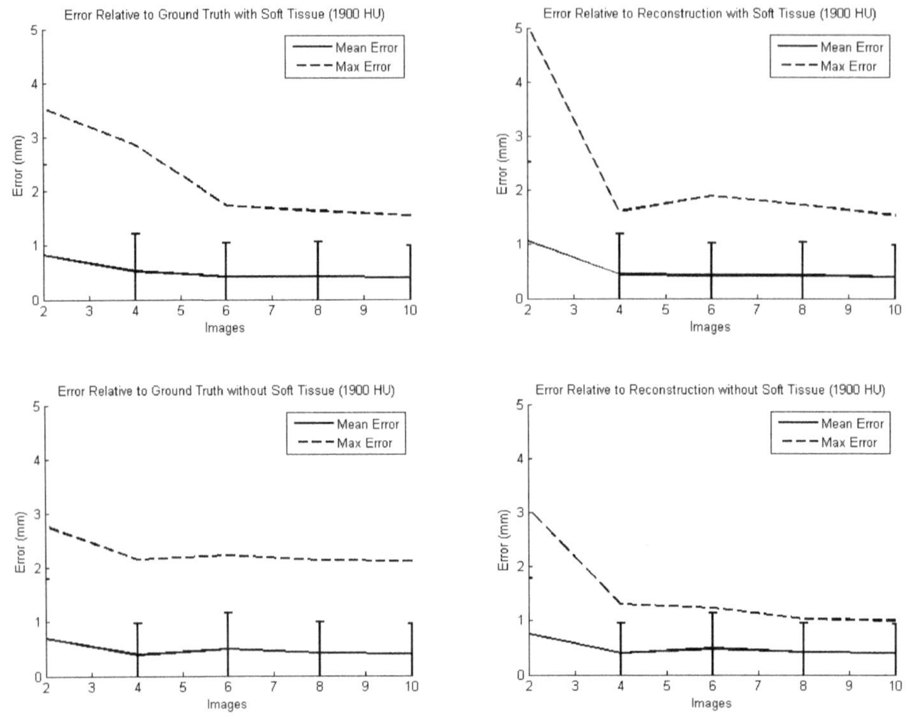

Fig. 6. Error between ground truth and SxMAC reconstruction for different numbers of X-Ray images. Error bars indicate one standard deviation from the mean.

error for reconstruction-to-truth and truth-to-reconstruction of 2 mm and 0.77 mm respectively. The CBCT and deformable model's level set representation were sampled at 1 mm isotropic. The background $\omega_{bg}(\boldsymbol{X})$ corresponded to a segmentation of the femur. In the first experiment, the attenuation of the cement was varied from 1645 HU to 2070 HU at equal intervals, and the number of images was held constant at 4 images (Fig. 5). In the second experiment, the number of images was varied from 2 to 10. Each collection of images was evenly sampled in plane from a 180° arc trajectory. The cement's attenuation was held constant at 1900 HU (Fig. 6). Pre-operative reconstruction errors were measured in terms of distance between mesh vertices on the ground truth and reconstructed surface.

5 Discussion

Results demonstrate SxMAC's ability to use intensity information to recover shape information that is not recoverable with silhouette reconstruction alone. Results from the cadaver experiment demonstrate SxMAC's reconstruction performance with prior CT. Fig. 5 suggests SxMAC reconstruction can be greatly improved by increasing the bone cement attenuation from 1550 HU to at least 1900 HU. An increase in attenuation could be achieved by using a higher concentration of Barium in the

PMMA bone cement. Fig. 6 demonstrates sub-millimeter accuracy is achievable with 4 images, and there is no significant improvement in accuracy for more than 8 images. Acquisition of 4 to 8 images is clinically relevant for intra-operative procedures. SxMAC is more sensitive to changes in contrast than the number of images, especially in the presence of soft-tissue.

In the absence of a shape prior for bone cement, SxMAC compensates by using a strong appearance prior derived from pre-operative CT. Performance is bolstered by SxMAC's use of silhouette reconstruction to provide an accurate initial estimate for the object's shape and appearance, which improves robustness and accelerates the algorithm's convergence.

There are other ways to model prior information observed in X-Rays. For instance, a prior model of a patient's anatomy (i.e. pelvis or femur) can be registered to X-Rays. After which, the anatomy can be removed from the image by a DRR/X-Ray differencing technique [18]. If the object of interest is a bone, Dual-X-Ray Absorptionmetry (DXA) imaging can be used to remove the appearance of soft-tissue in X-Ray images [19]. DXA images may be more appropriate for bone cement reconstruction because experiments demonstrate SxMAC performs better in the absence of soft tissue.

The synthesized X-Ray images used to evaluate SxMAC are representative of ideal results achievable with the following pre-processing pipeline: register the diagnostic CT to X-Ray images, generate DRRs from diagnostic CT, and remap the X-Ray intensities to DRR intensities. SxMAC's true performance during an intra-operative procedure will be affected by the performance of these pre-processing steps.

6 Conclusion

This paper has presented an algorithm for 3D segmentation of bone cement observed in a small number of X-Ray images. The SxMAC algorithm provides a computationally efficient procedure for segmentation that can incorporate prior CT and an initial estimate for the object's shape and location. The algorithm is implemented within an automated pipeline whose inputs are pre-processed X-Rays, their associated pose information, and prior CT, if available. A cadaver experiment demonstrates SxMAC can segment injected bone cement with sub-millimeter accuracy from as few as 4 X-Ray images and thus readily applicable to intra-operative surgical procedures.

Acknowledgments. This research has been financially supported by NIH grant 5R21EB007747-02, a graduate student fellowship from the Johns Hopkins Applied Physics Laboratory, and a research fellowship from JSPS Postdoctoral Fellowships for Research Abroad.

References

1. Sadowsky, O., et al.: Hybrid Cone-Beam Tomographic Reconstruction: Incorporation of Prior Anatomical Models to Compensate for Missing Data. IEEE Transactions on Medical Imaging 30(1), 69–83 (2011)

2. Garfin, S.R., Yuan, H.A., Reiley, M.A.: New technologies in spine: kyphoplasty and vertebroplasty for the treatment of painful osteoporotic compression fractures. Spine 26(14), 1511 (2001)
3. Richards, A., et al.: Biomechanical Analysis of Sacroplasty: Does Volume or Location of Cement Matter? American Journal of Neuroradiology 30(2), 315 (2009)
4. Beckmann, J., et al.: Femoroplasty-augmentation of the proximal femur with a composite bone cement-feasibility, biomechanical properties and osteosynthesis potential. Medical Engineering & Physics 29(7), 755–764 (2007)
5. Otake, Y., et al.: An image-guided femoroplasty system: development and initial cadaver studies. In: SPIE, San Diego, CA (2010)
6. Basafa, E., Armiger, R., Kutzer, M., Sutter, E., Mears, S., Armand, M.: Optimizing Cement Injection in Osteoporotic Femur Augmentation. In: Proc. of the 9th Annu. Meeting of CAOS-International 2009, Boston, MA (2009)
7. Laurentini, A.: The visual hull concept for silhouette-based image understanding. IEEE Trans. Pattern Analysis and Machine Intelligence, 150–162 (1994)
8. Liebschner, M., Templeton, A.: Intra-operative 3-D reconstruction of bone cement boli using X-rays, William Marsh Rice University (2009)
9. Kutulakos, K., Seitz, S.: A theory of shape by space carving. International Journal of Computer Vision 38(3), 199–218 (2000)
10. Caselles, V., Kimmel, R., Sapiro, G.: Geodesic active contours. International Journal of Computer Vision 22(1), 61–79 (1997)
11. Yezzi, A., Soatto, S.: Stereoscopic segmentation. International Journal of Computer Vision 53(1), 31–43 (2003)
12. Sadowsky, O.: Image registration and hybrid volume reconstruction of bone anatomy using a statistical shape atlas. Computer Science. Johns Hopkins University, Baltimore (2009)
13. Alvino, C., Yezzi, A.: Tomographic reconstruction of piecewise smooth images. IEEE Computer Society, Los Alamitos (2004); (1999)
14. Varshney, K., et al.: Multi-view stereo reconstruction of total knee replacement from X-rays. IEEE Trans. on Medical Image Analysis (2009)
15. Keil, A., Vogel, J., Lauritsch, G., Navab, N.: Dynamic cone beam reconstruction using a new level set formulation. In: Yang, G.-Z., Hawkes, D., Rueckert, D., Noble, A., Taylor, C., et al. (eds.) MICCAI 2009. LNCS, vol. 5762, pp. 389–397. Springer, Heidelberg (2009)
16. Yoon, S., Pineda, A., Fahrig, R.: Simultaneous segmentation and reconstruction: A level set method approach for limited view computed tomography. Medical Physics 37, 2329
17. Daly, M., et al.: Geometric calibration of a mobile C-arm for intraoperative cone-beam CT. Medical Physics 35, 2124 (2008)
18. Sadowsky, O.: Image registration and hybrid volume reconstruction of bone anatomy using a statistical shape atlas. Computer Science. Johns Hopkins University, Baltimore (2009)
19. Mazess, R., et al.: Dual-energy x-ray absorptiometry for total-body and regional bone-mineral and soft-tissue composition. American Journal of Clinical Nutrition 51(6), 1106 (1990)

Biomechanically Constrained Groupwise Statistical Shape Model to Ultrasound Registration of the Lumbar Spine

Siavash Khallaghi[1], Parvin Mousavi[2], Dan Borschneck[2], Gabor Fichtinger[2], and Purang Abolmaesumi[1]

[1] University of British Columbia, Vancouver, BC, Canada
[2] Queen's University, Kingston, ON, Canada
purang@ece.ubc.ca

Abstract. Spinal needle injections for back pain management are frequently carried out in hospitals and radiological clinics. Currently, these procedures are performed under fluoroscopy or CT guidance in specialized interventional radiology facilities. As an alternative, the use of inexpensive ultrasound image guidance promises to reduce the costs and increase the availability and safety of procedure. We propose to eliminate the need for ionizing radiation by creating a statistical shape model of the lumbar vertebrae and registering it to 3D ultrasound volumes of patient using a groupwise registration algorithm. From a total of 35 patient CT volumes, statistical shape models of the L2, L3 and L4 vertebrae are created, including the mean shapes and principal modes of variation. The statistical shape models are simultaneously registered to the 3D ultrasound by interchangeably optimizing the model parameters and their relative poses. We also use a biomechanical model to constrain the relative motion of the individual vertebra models throughout the registration process. The proposed method was validated on three phantoms with realistic spinal curvatures.

1 Introduction

Facet joint injection, a common percutaneous spinal injection procedure for pain management, requires an experienced physician to deliver the anesthetics to the target area. Contemporary approach to needle guidance with CT and fluoroscopy necessitates specialized facilities often unavailable to patients living in rural areas, and involves X-ray radiation. In contrast to CT and fluoroscopy, ultrasound (US) guidance has been considered, which is an accessible, portable, and non-ionizing imaging modality. For facet joint injections, Watson *et al.* [13] and Klocke *et al.* [9] targeted the L2-L3 and L3-L4 interspaces, a challenging procedure that, if performed inaccurately, damages the spinal cord. The results presented in both papers suggest that US as a mono-modal guidance is inadequate. To address this issue, the combination of US with CT has been proposed in an inter-modality registration framework [5,10,15].

Accurate registration of US and CT images has proven to be a challenging problem because of the low Signal to Noise Ratio (SNR) of US images and the

R.H. Taylor and G.-Z. Yang (Eds.): IPCAI 2011, LNCS 6689, pp. 47–54, 2011.

presence of artifacts. Hence, most of the existing algorithms preprocess either of the modalities to reduce the artifacts and to increase the similarity between the images. Recently, Wein *et al.* [14] proposed to dynamically simulate US images from CT data using the physical properties of ultrasound. The simulated image is updated throughout the registration process until a correct alignment is achieved between the US and CT.

Many groups have considered Statistical Shape Models (SSMs) [2] as an alternative to preoperative CT scans [1,3]. In this framework, prior knowledge of the anatomy is introduced through the SSM, which removes the need for CT scans. Talib *et al.* [11] investigated the feasibility of US registration to SSMs of the femur. Barratt *et al.* [1] and Foroughi *et al.* [3] built SSMs for the femur and pelvis, which are subsequently repositioned and deformed to fit a cloud of bone surface points extracted from a set of tracked US images. All the above approaches require preprocessing of US data to highlight the location of bone surface. Previously, we demonstrated the feasibility of US registration to SSM of a single vertebra [8] without the need for prior segmentation of US images.

For facet joint injections, using SSMs to guide the intervention is ideal, as normally, preoperative CTs are not available. As facet joints are located at the intersection of two vertebrae, SSM of more than one vertebra has to be registered to US images. In addition, the significant occlusion of adjacent vertebrae in US data makes the single SSM to US registration approach challenging. To alleviate this problem, we propose the first report of the simultaneous registration of multiple vertebrae SSMs to US. The extension of the problem from single SSM [8] to multiple SSMs is nontrivial, as the number of parameters to be optimized grows exponentially with the addition of each SSM. To constrain the possible solutions for the registration problem, we incorporate a biomechanical model of spine motion [4]. In phantom experiments, we demonstrate improved registration results and higher success rates in comparison to the single SSM registration approach [8].

2 Methodology

2.1 CT Data Collection

The CT data were collected at a local hospital under the approval of the Research Ethics Board. A set of CT images, acquired from 38 patients (19 male and 19 female), was used where the L2, L3 and L4 vertebrae were semi-automatically segmented using ITK-Snap [16] and resampled into $120 \times 200 \times 100$ voxels with an isotropic spacing of 0.6 mm. The patient data was divided into two groups: 35 for constructing the SSM (hereafter referred to as training data), and three for validation (two male and one female).

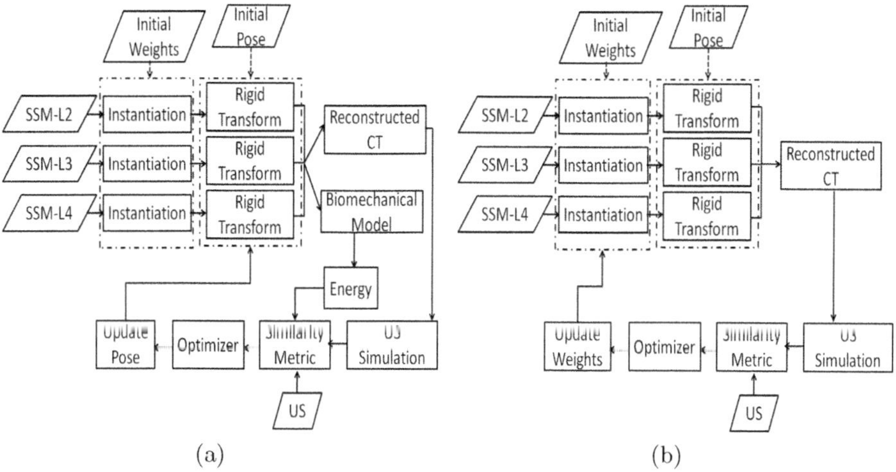

Fig. 1. Detailed description of the (a) rigid and (b) deformable registration blocks for groupwise registration

2.2 Statistical Shape Model Construction

To construct the SSM for each vertebra, we use the approach we have proposed previously [8]. For each SSM, a patient CT volume close to the mean shape of the population is chosen as the template. Each training example is registered to the template by a rigid registration followed by a B-spline deformable registration. With the deformable transformation of all the training examples known with respect to the template, principal component analysis (PCA) is performed to construct the SSM.

Individual vertebra SSMs are used to generate new instances of the population. Each instance is produced by a linear combination of the mean deformation vector, SSM weights, and the eigenvectors of the covariance matrix generated from all the deformation fields. The SSM weights provide a compact description of the transformation needed to deform the mean shape into the shape of the new instance. In our case the first 12 eigenvectors cover 95% of variations in shape for each vertebra.

2.3 Groupwise Registration

This section describes the SSM to US registration method for the L2, L3 and L4 vertebrae. The registration problem is solved in two steps: first rigid and then deformable. At the rigid stage, starting from 18 random initial rigid parameters (six for each vertebra, i.e. the pose) and zero SSM weights, the algorithm solves for the optimal rigid parameters. Subsequently, at the deformable stage, the algorithm finds 36 optimal deformable parameters (12 for each vertebra, i.e. the SSM weights). Using the updated rigid and deformable parameters, the algorithm iterates through the rigid and deformable phases until convergence is achieved. For optimization, Covariance Matrix Adaptation Evolution Strategy (CMA-ES) is used as optimizer because it yields convergence in a irregular search space [15]. Decoupling the problem into rigid and deformable registration phases, not only decreases the complexity of the problem, but also allows for a faster convergence by decreasing the population size of the CMA-ES optimizer.

The rigid registration phase is shown in Figure 1(a). First, we set the initial SSM weights to zero, and generate an instance of each of the L2, L3 and L4 vertebrae. Then, using a random initial rigid transformation, each generated instance is perturbed to an initial pose. After the rigid transformations are applied, the instances are reconstructed into a single volume. For any overlapping voxels, the maximum intensity is selected, thus preserving bone structure. Any gaps in the final volume are filled with a default value approximating the intensity of soft tissue in CT. Then, a ray-casting based ultrasound simulation is applied to the reconstructed volume. Assuming that the Hounsfield units can be related to the acoustic impedance values used to calculate ultrasound transmission and reflection, each ultrasound beam is modelled as a ray passing down the columns of the image [14]. Next, the Linear Correlation of Linear Combination (LC^2) metric is calculated and is fused with a biomechanical model to produce the final similarity measure. This similarity measure is fed to the CMA-ES optimizer until all of rigid parameters converge. A similar approach is employed for the groupwise deformable registration phase, as shown in Figure 1(b). The registration iterates between deformable and rigid phases until the correct pose and shape of the SSMs are found.

2.4 Biomechanical Model

For multiple SSM to US registration, the search space of the parameters to be optimized is relatively large, making convergence to a global minimum challenging. In addition, allowing free motion of the vertebrae during the course of the groupwise registration may result in anatomically unrealistic alignments where the vertebrae are in invalid orientations, colliding or far apart. In order to constrain the space of possible registration outcomes, a biomechanical model [5] is employed. Using a stiffness matrix, this model constrains the vertebrae to a common rotational orientation with no translation perpendicular to the sagittal and coronal planes. The total energy of the system, E, is calculated for all the vertebrae and normalized with respect to the maximum misalignment energy that is generated by 10 mm translation along the axes and 10 degrees about each axis. This normalized energy is incorporated in the computation of the image similarity metric, Biomechanically Constrained Linear Correlation of Linear Combinations ($BCLC^2$):

$$BCLC^2 = LC^2 - \sigma E \quad (1)$$

where σ is a constant that determines the contribution of the biomechanical model. In our case, we used a value of 0.75, previously found to be optimum in terms of registration success rate [5].

3 Experiments and Results

3.1 Ultrasound Data Acquisition

As mentioned in subsection 2.1, we excluded three CT volumes from the patient data for validation. We constructed 3D models of L1 to L5 vertebrae of these patients and printed them using a Cimetrix 3D shape printer (Cimetrix Solutions, Oshawa, ON, Canada). Three spine phantoms were constructed by submerging the models in an agar-gelatine-based gel. A high-resolution CT image ($0.46 \times 0.46 \times 0.625$ mm) and an ultrasound volume were acquired from each phantom from a freehand sweep using a tracked L14-5/38 linear-array transducer and a Sonix RP ultrasound machine (Ultrasonix, Richmond, BC, Canada) operating at 6.6 MHz with an imaging depth of 5.5 cm. Nine fiducial markers, mounted on the exterior of the phantom box, were localized with a tracked pointer and transformed to US space. The CT and ultrasound volumes were aligned using these markers.

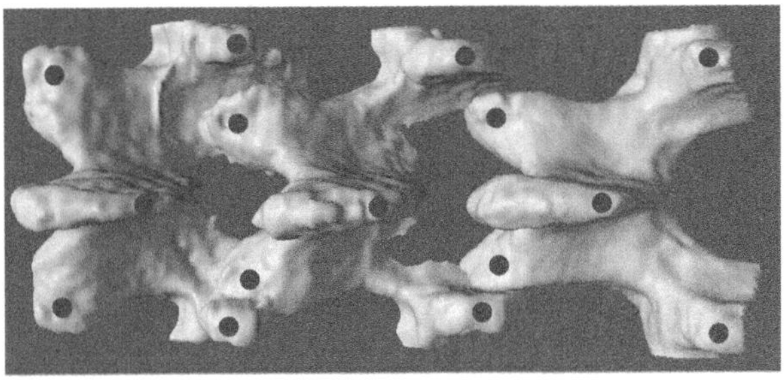

Fig. 2. The red circles mark the position of the surgeon-selected landmarks on the surface of the vertebrae

3.2 Results

The SSMs of the L2, L3 and L4 were brought to an initial pose by a rigid registration between the mean instance and the corresponding phantom CT volume. Then the groupwise SSM to US registration was performed. For each phantom, a total of 30 experiments were performed starting from a random position and orientation about the initial pose. This random perturbation was generated using a uniform distribution in the [0,10] mm translation along each anatomical axis and $[0,10]^\circ$ rotation about each axis.

An expert orthopaedic surgeon was asked to identify 15 anatomical landmarks on the surface of the superior and inferior articular process of each vertebra on the registered SSM, the ultrasound and the corresponding CT volume, as illustrated in Figure 2. The average distance of the five landmarks on the registered SSM and the corresponding CT was chosen as a measure of the final Target Registration Error (TRE), as it was harder for the physician to establish correspondence between the US and the registered SSM. The groupwise registration

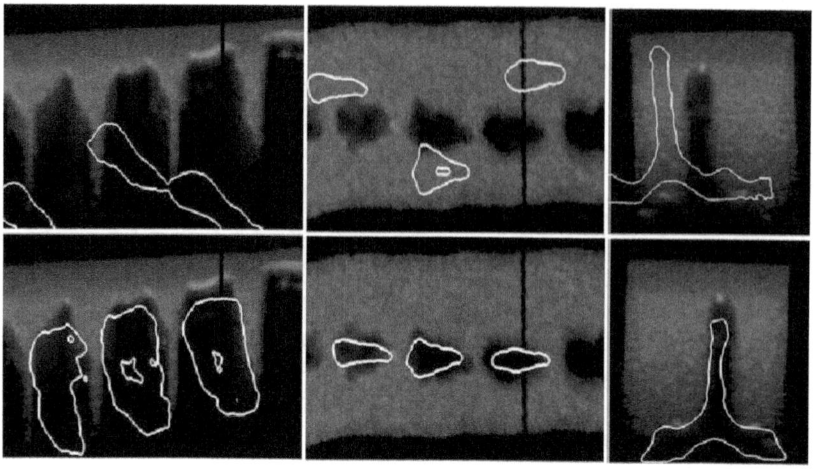

Fig. 3. Transverse (left), coronal (center), and sagittal (right) slices of the original ultrasound volume overlayed with the bone contours of the misaligned (top) and groupwise registered (bottom) SSM volumes

is considered to be successful, only if the final TRE for each vertebra was less than 3.0 mm, a clinically acceptable error tolerance for facet joint injections [5]. The Success Rate (SR), mean, standard deviation and the final TRE for the 30 experiments for each phantom are shown in Table 1. Success rate is defined as the ratio of successful results over the total number of registrations. Individual success rate for each vertebra and also the Group Success Rate (GSR) for all vertebrae are reported. A registration is considered as successful only if the final TRE is less than 3.0 mm for each vertebra. Figure 3 shows the overlay of the registered SSMs of L2, L3 and L4 with the ultrasound volume, prior to and following registration.

Table 1. Results for the SSM to ultrasound groupwise registration

	L2			L3			L4			
Phantom	Mean	STD	SR	Mean	STD	SR	Mean	STD	SR	GSR
1	2.49	0.49	79%	2.56	0.33	82%	2.36	0.43	79%	79%
2	2.40	0.41	70%	2.41	0.29	75%	2.36	0.43	70%	70%
3	2.43	0.36	75%	2.4	0.34	82%	2.56	0.33	75%	75%

As seen in Table 1, the groupwise registration method resulted in an average success rate of 70% with the average TRE below 3 mm for the successful cases. The landmark errors for successful cases were below 3 mm, which is a sufficiently close distance to envelope the nerve sack in the anesthetic agent without endangering the spinal cord. Comparing the results with Khallaghi *et al.* [8] shows that the mean TRE for all vertebrae is well below the threshold of 3 mm, while the overall success rate stays high. This is expected since the neighbouring vertebrae constrain the set of solutions for the registration.

Several factors limit the success rate of the groupwise registration. Due to partial volume occlusion, it is impossible to visualize the superior articular process in ultrasound images. Also, creating an instant of the SSM to capture the sharp corners of the spinous and transverse processes is a challenging task. While the former is intrinsic to ultrasound imaging, the latter can be substantially improved by increasing the number of training images and using a denser grid in the construction of the SSM.

The template CT chosen to create the SSM is from a patient close to the mean shape of the population. This may introduce a bias in SSM towards the template, which may result in larger registration errors when the patient anatomy is far from the template. To avoid this problem, we will consider using unbiased, template-free, techniques to create the SSM in future research [7,12].

The proposed registration method shows promise in the phantom experiments; there are certain challenges to overcome in order to translate it to a clinical setting: 1) The signature of the vertebrae in US images of human is substantially different from the phantom data in terms of the speckle pattern and the visibility of vertebrae surfaces due to the loss of signal and strong reflections caused by surrounding anatomy. Our preliminary results from *ex vivo* experiments on lamb cadavers demonstrate the feasibility of accurate registration between 3D US images and CT data of lumbar spine [4]. Accordingly, we expect that with reasonably accurate initial alignment of the SSM and 3D US, the proposed technique will converge in human data. In other words, the error ranges will be comparable to this study, but the capture range will be limited. A graphical user interface will be required to select corresponding anatomical regions in SSM and US data to obtain the initial alignment. 2) The current runtime for the proposed method is in the order of hours, the bottleneck being the instance generation. By implementing the instantiation on a Graphics Processing Unit (GPU), a significant improvement in runtime is possible [6].

Acknowledgements

This work was funded by the Natural Sciences and Engineering Research Council of Canada (NSERC) and the Canadian Institutes of Health Research (CIHR).

References

1. Barratt, D.C., Chan, C.S.K., Edwards, P.J., Penney, G.P., Slomczykowski, M., Carter, T.J., Hawkes, D.J.: Instantiation and registration of statistical shape models of the femur and pelvis using 3d ultrasound imaging. Medical Image Analysis 12(3), 358–374 (2008)
2. Cootes, T.F., Taylor, C.J., Cooper, D.H., Graham, J.: Active shape models their training and application. Computer Vision and Image Understanding 61(1), 38–59 (1995)

3. Foroughi, P., Song, D., Chintalapani, G., Taylor, R.H., Fichtinger, G.: Localization of pelvic anatomical coordinate system using uS/Atlas registration for total hip replacement. In: Metaxas, D., Axel, L., Fichtinger, G., Székely, G. (eds.) MICCAI 2008, Part II. LNCS, vol. 5242, pp. 871–879. Springer, Heidelberg (2008)
4. Gill, S., Abolmaesumi, P., Fichtinger, G., Boisvert, J., Pichora, D., Borschneck, D., Mousavi, P.: Biomechanically constrained groupwise ultrasound to ct registration of the lumbar spine. Medical Image Analysis (2010) (in press)
5. Gill, S., Mousavi, P., Fichtinger, G., Chen, E., Boisvert, J., Pichora, D., Abolmaesumi, P.: Biomechanically constrained groupwise US to CT registration of the lumbar spine. In: Yang, G.-Z., Hawkes, D., Rueckert, D., Noble, A., Taylor, C. (eds.) MICCAI 2009. LNCS, vol. 5761, pp. 803–810. Springer, Heidelberg (2009)
6. Gong, R.H., Stewart, J., Abolmaesumi, P.: A new representation of intensity atlas for gpu-accelerated instance generation. In: 2010 Annual International Conference of the IEEE Engineering in Medicine and Biology Society (EMBC), August 31-September 4, pp. 4399–4402 (2010)
7. Joshi, S., Davis, B., Jomier, M., Gerig, G.: Unbiased diffeomorphic atlas construction for computational anatomy. NeuroImage 23(1), 151–160 (2004)
8. Khallaghi, S., Mousavi, P., Gong, R.H., Gill, S., Boisvert, J., Fichtinger, G., Pichora, D., Borschneck, D., Abolmaesumi, P.: Registration of a statistical shape model of the lumbar spine to 3D ultrasound images. In: Jiang, T., Navab, N., Pluim, J.P.W., Viergever, M.A. (eds.) MICCAI 2010. LNCS, vol. 6362, pp. 68–75. Springer, Heidelberg (2010)
9. Klocke, R., Jenkinson, T., Glew, D.: Sonographically guided caudal epidural steroid injections. Journal of Ultrasound in Medicine 22(11), 1229–1232 (2003)
10. Moore, J., Clarke, C., Bainbridge, D., Wedlake, C., Wiles, A., Pace, D., Peters, T.: Image guidance for spinal facet injections using tracked ultrasound. In: Yang, G.-Z., Hawkes, D., Rueckert, D., Noble, A., Taylor, C. (eds.) MICCAI 2009. LNCS, vol. 5761, pp. 516–523. Springer, Heidelberg (2009)
11. Talib, H., Rajamani, K., Kowal, J., Nolte, L.P., Styner, M., Ballester, M.A.G.: A comparison study assessing the fesibility of ultrasound-initialized deformable bone models. Computer Aided Surgery 10(5/6), 293–299 (2005)
12. Wang, Q., Chen, L., Yap, P., et al.: Groupwise registration based on hierarchical image clustering and atlas synthesis. Human Brain Mapping 31(8), 1128–1140 (2010)
13. Watson, M.J., Evans, S., Thorp, J.M.: Could ultrasonography be used by an anaesthetist to identify a specified lumbar interspace before spinal anaesthesia? British Journal of Anaesthesia 90(4), 509–511 (2003)
14. Wein, W., Brunke, S., Khamene, A., Callstrom, M.R., Navab, N.: Automatic ct-ultrasound registration for diagnostic imaging and image-guided intervention. Medical Image Analysis 12(5), 577–585 (2008)
15. Winter, S., Brendel, B., Pechlivanis, I., Schmieder, K., Igel, C.: Registration of CT and intraoperative 3D ultrasound images of the spine using evolutionary and gradient-based methods. IEEE Transactions on Evolutionary Computation 12(3), 284–296 (2008)
16. Yushkevich, P.A., Piven, J., Cody Hazlett, H., Gimpel Smith, R., Ho, S., Gee, J.C., Gerig, G.: User-guided 3D active contour segmentation of anatomical structures: Significantly improved efficiency and reliability. Neuroimage 31(3), 1116–1128 (2006)

Visual Tracking of Surgical Tools for Proximity Detection in Retinal Surgery

Rogério Richa, Marcin Balicki, Eric Meisner, Raphael Sznitman, Russell Taylor, and Gregory Hager

Laboratory for Computational Science and Robotics (LCSR)
Johns Hopkins University, Baltimore MD, USA
{richa,marcin,meisner,sznitman,rht,hager}@jhu.edu

Abstract. In retinal surgery, surgeons face difficulties such as indirect visualization of surgical targets, physiological tremor and lack of tactile feedback. Such difficulties increase the risks of incorrect surgical gestures which may cause retinal damage. In this context, robotic assistance has the potential to overcome current technical limitations and increase surgical safety. In this paper we present a method for robustly tracking surgical tools in retinal surgery for detecting proximity between surgical tools and the retinal surface. An image similarity function based on weighted mutual information is specially tailored for tracking under critical illumination variations, lens distortions, and rapid motion. The proposed method was tested on challenging conditions using a phantom eye and recorded human *in vivo* data acquired by an ophthalmic stereo microscope.

Keywords: visual tracking, mutual information, robotic assisted retinal surgery.

1 Introduction

Sight-threatening conditions such as retinal detachment and macular holes currently require technically challenging surgical interventions. Surgeons face several difficulties, starting with the indirect visualization of the surgical targets, hand tremor and lack of tactile feedback. In recent years, first generation smart sensing tools have been developed in order to overcome some of the challenges in retinal surgery. Examples are the micro force sensor in [1] and optical coherence tomography instrument described in [2]. However, current sensors require tools to be in contact or very close to the retinal surface, increasing the risk of unintentional collisions with the delicate intra-ocular tissue. Furthermore, in robotic assisted vitreoretinal surgery, the end-effector kinematics are also difficult to estimate due to the very thin, long and relatively flexible instruments.

In this context, computer vision techniques have the potential of providing contactless proximity detection, complementing previously developed smart tools. To this end, accurate visual tracking of surgical tools in microscopic images is required. In the literature, several works on surgical tool tracking exist and they can be coarsely categorised into two classes [3]: color-based and

R.H. Taylor and G.-Z. Yang (Eds.): IPCAI 2011, LNCS 6689, pp. 55–66, 2011.

geometry-based approaches. In color-based approaches [4,5,6], tools are detected and tracked based on the color information on the images and artificial markers are often employed. On the other hand, geometry-based appproaches are based on the tool shape [7,8]. Although tracking based on geometry information is more challenging than color-based tracking, issues concerning bio-compatibility and sterilisability due to the use of color markers can be avoided.

In this paper we propose a robust method for visually tracking surgical tools with a novel image similarity measure based on weighted mutual information. The novel similarity measure has the advantage of being robust to illumination variations, lens distortions and partial occlusions. The proposed tool tracking method is evaluated through several experiments using recorded images of a custom made phantom eye and human *in vivo* data. The method is also tested in a proximity detection task, demonstrating its potential for increasing surgical safety.

This paper is organized as follows. In the next section we discuss the main challenges of tracking a surgical tool in microscopic images and describe the novel similarity function based on weighted mutual information used in our work. In section 3, we evaluate the performance of the proposed tracking method under large illumination variations, partial occlusions and rapid motion. Finally, we tested the proposed tool tracking method in a proximity detection task and conclude the paper in section 4.

2 Materials and Methods

The challenges involved in tracking surgical instruments start with the illumination conditions during surgery. Surgeons often use a hand-held light pipe to illuminate the retina (Figure 1), causing lighting to be irregular and highly variable between frames. Exterior lighting (from the operating room) can also cause

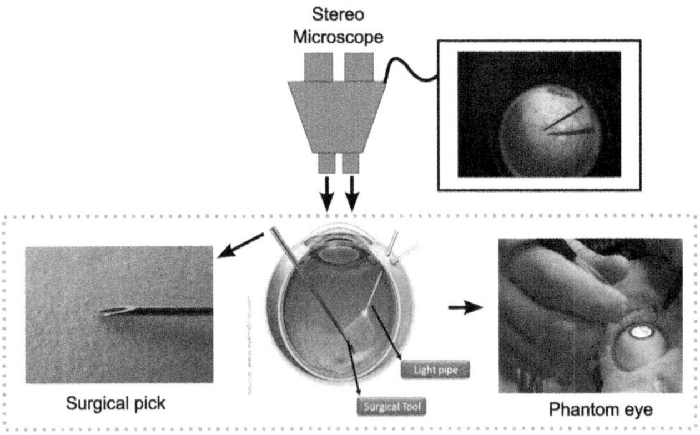

Fig. 1. Experimental setup (Bottom) Surgical tools inside the human eye and the eye phantom used in the experiments. (Top) Visualization through the microscope.

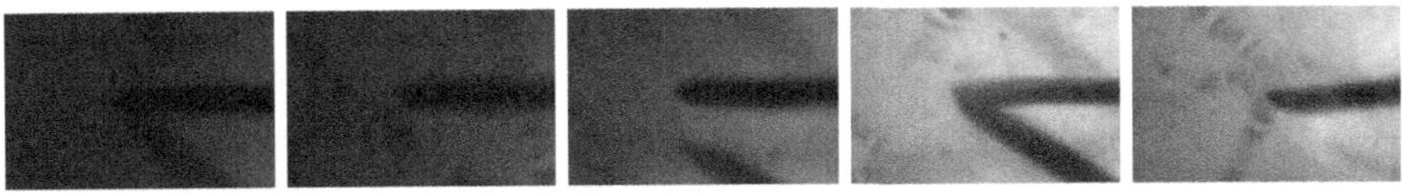

Fig. 2. Tracking a surgical tool Typical images of a surgical tool tip during experiments with an eye phantom

glares, further complicating the visual tracking task. In addition, image distortions caused by the eye and microscope lenses are difficult to correct for due to their complexity and variability (Figure 2).

An example of a pick tool used in current surgical practice is illustrated in Figure 1. Although it has a simple appearance model (i.e. a dark rectangular shaft), tracking based on standard image similarity measures (e.g. sum of squared distances [9], Matusita [10], normalized cross correlation, etc) fails due to the disturbances mentioned above. The limited choice of similarity measures suitable for this problem motivates the design of a measure based on mutual information specially tailored for overcoming the shortcomings of standard approaches.

2.1 Tracking Using Mutual Information

The tip of the surgical tool is tracked using a 3 DOF motion model (an Euclidean transformation). Since the stereo images are not calibrated, the tool tip is tracked separately on both stereo images from the microscope. Given a reference image of the tool tip, tracking is divided into two stages:

1. **Brute force search** - For every frame, we search for the new tool tip position in the neighborhood of the tool location in the previous frame. For computational reasons, the inter-frame rotational component is neglected in this step. This search is necessary for coping with large inter frame motions and its result is used for initializing a gradient-based optimization closer to the correct tool position. For the search, we use a novel measure based on weighted mutual information, which is presented in details in section 2.2.
2. **Gradient-based tracking** - For an accurate tool position estimation, the MI gradient-based tracking method proposed by Dame *et al.* [11] is employed. Details on its implementation are given in section 2.3.

2.2 Weighted Mutual Information

In the context of visual tracking, mutual information (MI) is a measure of the shared information between two images. It gives high scores for image pairs that share a sparse joint distribution. This has a very intuitive interpretation: a good match between two images occurs when darker pixels on one image align with darker pixels of the other, while bright pixels align with bright pixels. As a result, visual tracking based on MI is intrinsically invariant to non-linear illumination variations.

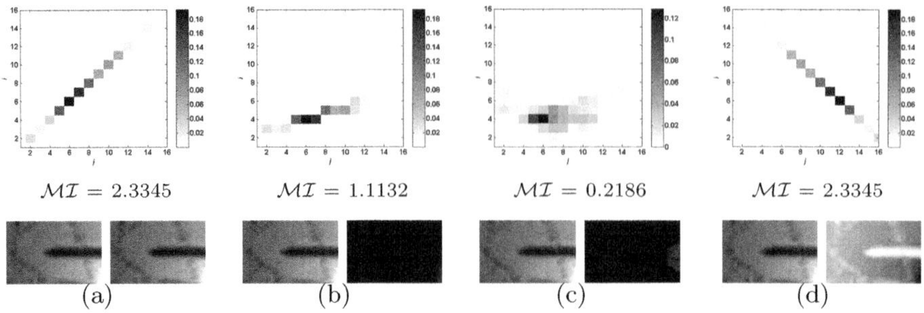

Fig. 3. Joint Intensity Distributions the x and y axes correspond to intensity bins of the reference and target images, respectively. (a) the joint distribution of an image with itself (b) illumination changes (c) misaligned images (d) an image with its inverse.

However, certain joint distribution configurations which are interpreted as good matches may not have any physical meaning in practice. Normally, when tracking using cameras it is not expected that bright pixels turn dark and dark pixels turn bright simultaneously. Although this flexibility is key for multi-modal image alignment [12], it produces undesirable results in visual tracking. For this reason, we propose to apply weights to constrain the shape of the joint intensity distribution, keeping the robustness towards non-linear illumination variations while eliminating false matches.

Given the joint intensity distribution $p_{\mathcal{TI}}$ between reference and target images $\mathbf{T}$ and $\mathbf{I}$, respectively, the MI between images is computed as:

$$\mathcal{MI}(\mu) = \sum_{j,i} p_{\mathcal{TI}}(j,i,\mu) \log \left(\frac{p_{\mathcal{TI}}(j,i,\mu)}{p_{\mathcal{T}}(j) p_{\mathcal{I}}(i,\mu)} \right) \tag{1}$$

where $(j,\ i)$ are intensity histogram bins corresponding to the reference and target image histograms $p_{\mathcal{T}}$ and $p_{\mathcal{I}}$, respectively, and μ is the parameter vector of the transformation model. In this study, we use 8-bit grayscale images divided in 16 intensity bins[1]. The joint intensity distribution $p_{\mathcal{TI}}$ can be computed as:

$$p_{\mathcal{TI}}(j,i,\mu) = \sum_{\mathbf{x}} \delta(j - T(\mathbf{x}))\delta(i - I(\mathbf{x},\mu)) \tag{2}$$

where $\mathbf{x}$ are pixel positions and the column and row axes correspond to pixel intensities of the reference and target images, respectively. When the reference and target images $\mathbf{T}$ and $\mathbf{I}$ align perfectly, their joint intensity distribution is concentrated on the diagonal elements (see Figure 3(a)). However, when images do not match, the joint distribution is spread (Figure 3(c)) and the MI score is relatively low. MI also gives high scores for shifts in the pixel intensities of the target image, which make the metric robust to non-linear illumination variations

[1] The choice for the number of bins is justified in section 3.1.

(Figure 3(b)). However, although distributions such as the one illustrated in Figure 3(d) obtain high similarity scores, they often make no sense in practice.

For this reason, we propose to weight equation (2) and restrain the joint distribution configurations:

$$p'_{TI}(j,i,\mu) = \sum_{\mathbf{x}} w(j,i)\,\delta(j - T(\mathbf{x}))\delta(i - I(\mathbf{x},\mu)) \quad (3)$$

where the weights $w(j,i)$ are defined by the composition of 1D kernel functions (one for each column j of the joint distribution), centered on the intensity value c_j with span σ:

$$w(i,j) = \alpha\, k_j(||\frac{i - c_j}{\sigma}||) \quad (4)$$

where α is a normalization constant and $k_j(s) = 1$ for $s \in [c_j - \sigma, c_j + \sigma]$ or 0 otherwise. Figure 4(a) shows an example of an 16×16 weighting matrix using a roof kernel with $c_j = j$ and $\sigma = 3$. Weighting the joint intensity distribution has the same effect of 'turning on and off' pixels and their contributions to the similarity function in equation (1).

In the context of visual tracking, illumination changes induce vertical shifts in the joint distribution elements. In the previous example, only the elements of the weight matrix close to the diagonal have non-zero values, meaning that the similarity function is only invariant to small illumination changes. Hence, in order to design a weight matrix that is both robust to large illumination changes and eliminates false matches, we make the kernel parameter c vary during tracking. The parameters are initialized with $c_j = j$ and during tracking, once a match is found, the parameters c are updated based on the current joint distribution. A simple criterion for rejecting an alignment such as in Figure 3(d) is to set $c_j < c_{j+1}$, forcing kernel centers only to increase as a function of the column index. This enforces a weight function that favors distributions such as that illustrated in Figure 3(a). An example extracted of a weighting matrix using this principle is shown in Figure 4(b).

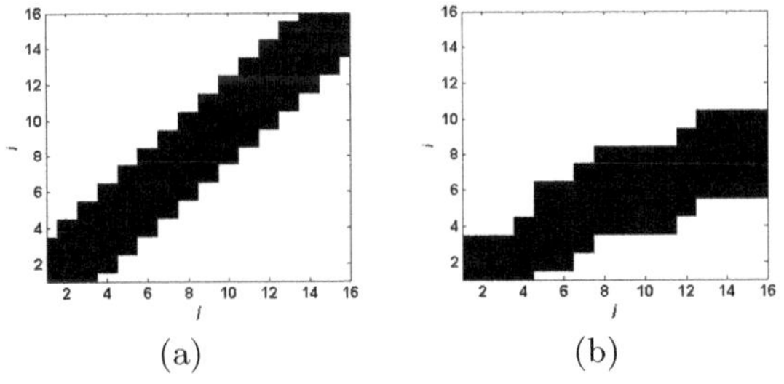

Fig. 4. Weight matrix (a) An example matrix $w(j,i)$ with $c_j = j$ and $\sigma = 3$. Dark and white elements are equal to 1 and 0 respectively. (b) An example of a weighting matrix during tracking. Notice the shape of the matrix adapts to shifts in the joint distribution caused by illumination variations similar to Figure 3(b).

2.3 Gradient-Based Mutual Information Tracking

Once the approximate position of the tool tip is found after a brute force search, the gradient-based mutual information tracking method proposed by Dame *et al.* [11] is applied.

Gradient-based methods [9] can achieve highly accurate results but they require a smooth convex similarity function. Therefore, it is first necessary to smooth the MI function from equation (1). In Dame *et al.* [11], this is achieved by smoothing the target image with a Gaussian kernel and using a kernel in the computation of the joint intensity histogram:

$$p^*_{TI}(j, i, \mu) = \sum_{\mathbf{x}} \phi(j - T(\mathbf{x}))\phi(i - I(\mathbf{x}, \mu)) \tag{5}$$

where $\phi(.)$ is a 3rd order B-spline function. In this manner, the MI function becomes smooth (even up to sub-pixel displacements) and an iterative optimization technique can then be applied for refining the tool tip position estimation. The optimal parameter vector μ for a given motion model is found by performing a second order Taylor expansion of equation (1) about μ is performed and setting its gradient to zero. The update $\Delta\mu$ for reaching the optimum is computed as:

$$\Delta\mu = -\mathbf{H}^{-1}\mathbf{G} \tag{6}$$

where $\mathbf{G}$ and $\mathbf{H}$ are the Gradient and Hessian matrices of the MI with respect to $\Delta\mu$:

$$\mathbf{G} = \frac{\partial \mathcal{MI}(I(\mathbf{x}, \mu), \mathbf{T}(\mathbf{x}))}{\partial \Delta\mu} \quad \mathbf{H} = \frac{\partial^2 \mathcal{MI}(I(\mathbf{x}, \mu), T(\mathbf{x}))}{\partial \Delta\mu^2} \tag{7}$$

Details on the computation of the equations above can be found in [11].

3 Experiments

The experimental validation of the tool tracking method is divided into two parts. First we perform an evaluation of the tool tracking performance with respect to illumination variations, partial occlusions and rapid motion. Second, we evaluate the proposed tracking method in a proximity detection task. All experiments were run off-line on recorded images using Matlab (MathWorks).

3.1 Tool Tracking

For acquiring images, we use two Point Grey cameras (Vancouver, Canada) coupled with the stereo microscope acquiring 1600x1200 pixel images at 30 fps. The images are transfered to the computer by FireWire and converted to 8-bit grayscale. Two sets of phantom image sequences and one set of images of a surgery performed on an *in vivo* human patient were recorded for the experiments.

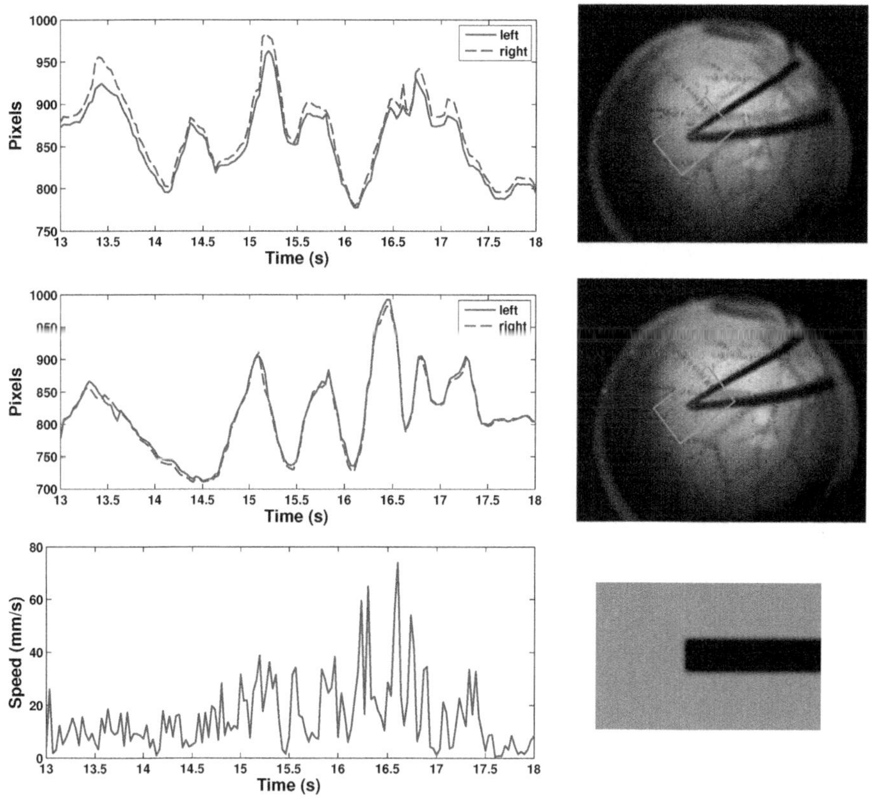

Fig. 5. Fast tool motions (top and middle left) the x and y coordinates of the tool displacement, in pixels, on left and right camera images. (bottom left) The approximate instantaneous tool speed inside the eye in [mm/s]. (top and middle right) Images of the left stereo camera corresponding to $t = 16.6s$ in (c). (bottom right) The reference image used for tracking in all phantom experiments.

Experiments with phantom data

The eye phantom is used to evaluate the performance of the proposed tool tracking method under three aspects: illumination variations, partial occlusions and fast tool motions. Since the tool tip appearance model is simple (a dark shaft on a bright background), we use the image in Figure 5(bottom right) as a reference image of the tool. This specific 200×150 pixel reference image is chosen according to the image resolution and it is designed to avoid possible tracking lock onto a specific background pattern. Since certain parts of the scene are poorly illuminated, 16 intensity bins were necessary in the computation of image histograms for keeping the discrimination between tool and background.

In the first image set, we manually move the tool inside the eye inducing rapid motion for testing the tracking robustness to large inter frame motion (Figure 5(top and middle right)). The set contains 580 images, acquired at 30

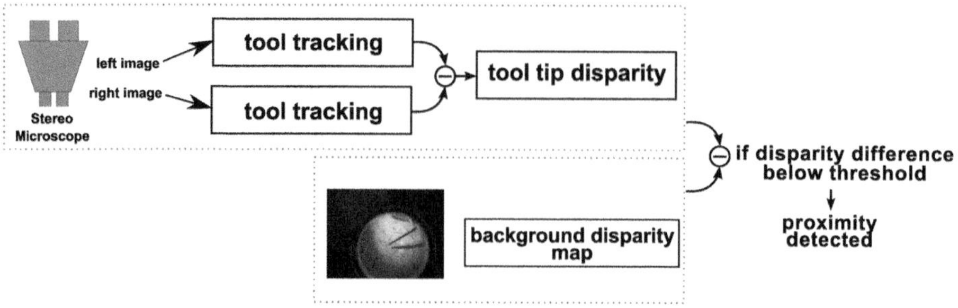

Fig. 6. Proximity detection A schematic overview of the proximity detection method

fps for 19.3s. In the brute force search step, we look for matches in a ±45 pixel neighborhood centered on the previous tool position. The displacement of the tool tip on both cameras is plotted in Figures 5(top and middle left). Given that the tool shaft diameter has 0.9 mm, we are also able to approximate the instantaneous tool speed inside the eye (Figure 5(bottom left)). Notice that speeds are considerably higher those observed in current surgical practice [2].

In the second image set, we track the tool under challenging illumination conditions (Figure 2). The set contains 520 images, acquired at 30 fps for 17.36s. Note that tracking is robust to occlusions caused by the tool shadow when the tool is close to the retinal surface.

Experiments with *in vivo* data

We applied the proposed tracking method on two sets of *in vivo* images of an inner limiting membrane (ILM) peeling procedure. The first set consists of images of the retina acquired with a wide-angle lens (Figure 7 top). In the second set, contact lenses for high-magnification are used (Figure 7 bottom). Even in the presence of large illumination variations, clutter and unmodeled changes in the tool appearance, the proposed tracking method is able to successfully retrieve the tool position on both image sets.

3.2 Proximity Detection

For demonstrating practical value in eye surgery, the proposed tool tracking method is tested in a proximity detection task. A diagram of the proposed system is shown in Figure 6. As mentioned in Section 2, since the stereo microscopic cameras are not calibrated, the tool tip is tracked separately on both stereo images. By considering only the vertical image disparities between the tool tip on the left and right images, we are able to avoid the complex task of modeling and identifying the microscope and eye lens distortion parameters. In this manner, proximity is detected when the difference between tool and background disparities is small.

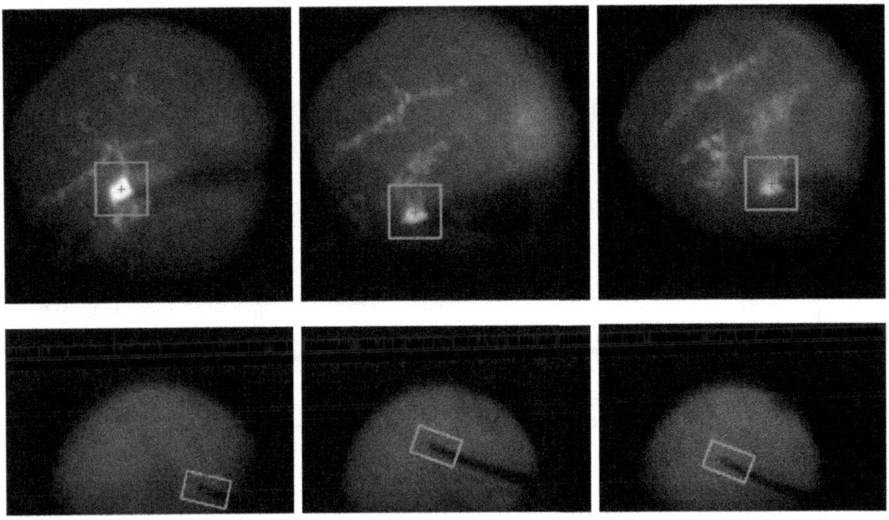

Fig. 7. In vivo tracking experiment (Top) The proposed method tracking the tip of a scrapping tool during an ILM peeling procedure. Notice the illumination changes as the tool moves away from the center of the field of view. Only the translational motion of the tool tip is tracked in this set due to its small size on the images. (Bottom) Tracking the tool on images acquired with a wide-angle lens.

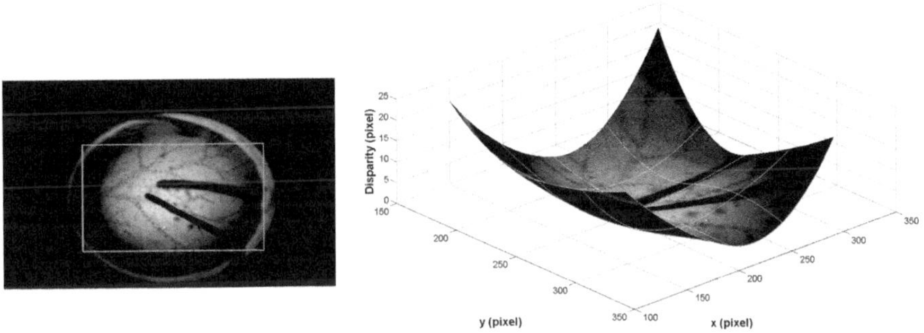

Fig. 8. Proximity detection A disparity map of the retinal surface is created using a B-spline deformable map with 16 control points evenly distributed on the reference image. Notice that the surgical tool is removed from the disparity map computation.

In our experiments we assume a static background (the eye phantom is fixed to the skull) and consider only the central region on the images where the estimation of the retinal surface disparity is not severely affected by lens distortions. Considering perspective distortions negligible, we compute a disparity map of the retina similar to [13] using a B-spline deformable map with 16 control points evenly distributed on a grid (see Figure 8). Notice that the surgical

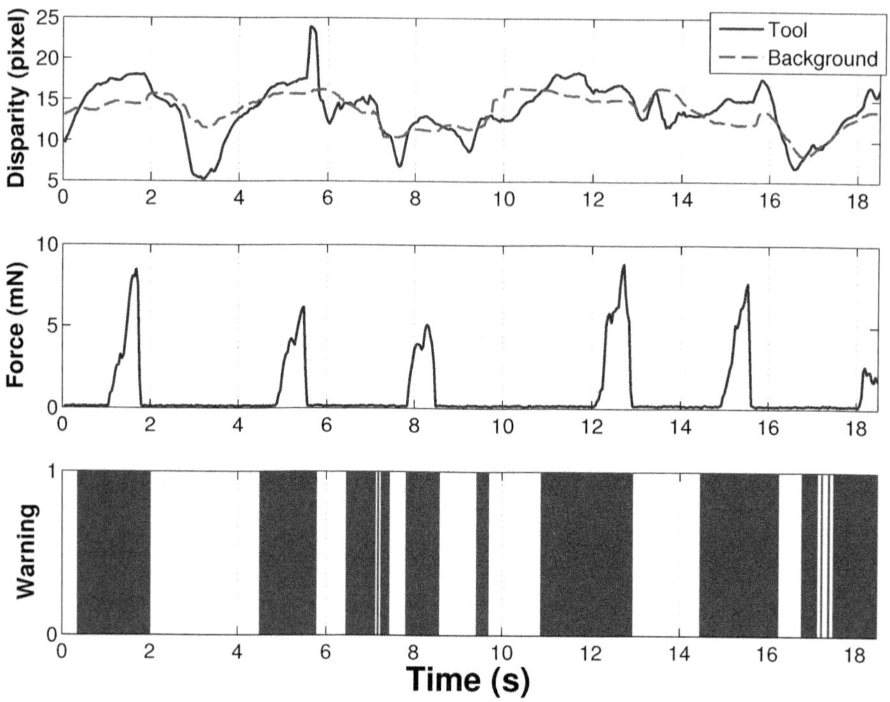

Fig. 9. Proximity detection (Top) The tool tip and relative background disparities. (Middle) The norm of forces applied on the tool shaft. (Bottom) Estimated proximity warnings estimated by the proposed method.

tool was removed from the image for the disparity map computation. In addition, the background is static and the disparity map is estimated only once for the whole experiment.

For comparing disparities between background and tool, the relative background disparity is extracted based on the tool position on the left camera image. The tool tip and relative background disparities are plotted in Figure 9(top). Due to imprecision in the disparity map estimation and the fact that we do not track the point of contact on the tool, the background and tool disparities are not equal when contact occurs. However, a proximity warning can be given a disparity difference smaller than 5 pixels (Figure 9(bottom)). This threshold was empirically given the diameter of the tool tip in the images. For assessing the detection efficiency, we used a surgical pick with a built-in 2DOF force sensor for providing ground-truth data. As expected, the force sensor readings (the norm of forces applied on the tool shaft) shown in Figure 9(middle) coincide with the proximity warnings given by the proposed proximity detection method. Since the tool often hovers the background at very close distances, many proximity alerts occur during the experiment.

4 Conclusion and Future Work

In this paper we propose a robust method for tracking surgical tools with an image similarity measure based on mutual information. The similarity metric used in our work has the advantage of being robust to rapid motion, illumination variations, lens distortions and partial occlusions due to shadows, as demonstrated by the experiments with the eye phantom. Furthermore, experiments with *in vivo* data attest the practical value of the proposed tracking method on a real clinical scenario. We have also demonstrated its potential for providing contactless proximity detection in retinal surgery for increased surgical safety.

We are currently working towards the incorporation of this capability into our robotic platform. Future work is concentrated on increasing the reliability of the proximity detection method by improving aspects such as the disparity map estimation and the automatic definition of safety limits.

Acknowledgements

The authors would like to thank Dr. Amaury Dame for the assistance and helpful comments. This work was partially supported by NIH Bioengineering Research Partnership grant NIH 1R01 EB007969.

References

1. Sun, Z., Balicki, M., Kang, J., Handa, J., Gehlbach, P., Taylor, R., Iordachita, I.: A sub-millimetric, 0.25 mn resolution fully integrated fiber-optic force sensing tool for retinal microsurgery. In: Proceedings of the International Congress on Computer Assisted Radiology and Surgery (CARS 2009), Berlin, Germany, pp. 383–390 (2009)
2. Balicki, M., Han, J.-H., Iordachita, I., Gehlbach, P., Handa, J., Taylor, R., Kang, J.: Single fiber optical coherence tomography microsurgical instruments for computer and robot-assisted retinal surgery. In: Yang, G.-Z., Hawkes, D., Rueckert, D., Noble, A., Taylor, C. (eds.) MICCAI 2009. LNCS, vol. 5761, pp. 108–115. Springer, Heidelberg (2009)
3. Groeger, M., Arbter, K., Hizinger, G.: Motion tracking for minimally invasive robotic surgery, pp. 117–148. I-Tech Education and Publishing (January 2008)
4. Wei, G.Q., Arbter, K., Hizinger, G.: Real-time visual servoing for laparoscopic surgery. In: Proceedings of IEEE International Conference of the Engineering in Medicine and Biology Society (EMBS 1997), Chicago, USA, pp. 40–45 (1997)
5. Tonet, O., Thoranaghatte, R., Megali, G., Dario, P.: Tracking endoscopic instruments without a localizer: a shape-analysis-based approach. Computer Aided Surgery 12(1), 35–42 (2007)
6. Doignon, C., Nagoette, F., de Mathelin, M.: Segmentation and guidance of multiple rigid objects for intra-operative endoscopic vision. In: Proceedings of the International Workshop on Dynamical Vision, in conjunction with ECCV 2006, Graz, Austria (2006)

7. Voros, S., Orvain, E., Long, J.-A., Cinquin, P.: Automatic detection of instruments in laparoscopic images: a first step towards high level command of robotized endoscopic holders. The International Journal of Robotics Research (IJRR) – Special Issue on Robot Vision 26(11-12), 119–173 (2007)
8. Pezzementi, Z., Voros, S., Hager, G.: Articulated object tracking by rendering consistent appearance parts. In: Proceedings of IEEE International Conference on Robotics and Automation (ICRA 2009), Kobe, Japan, pp. 3940–3947 (May 2009)
9. Baker, S., Matthews, I.: Lucas-kanade 20 years on: A unifying framework: Part 1. Technical report, Robotics Institute, Carnegie Mellon University, Pittsburgh, USA (July 2002)
10. Hager, G., Dewan, M., Stewart, C.: Multiple kernel tracking with ssd. In: Proceedings of IEEE Conference on Computer Vision and Pattern Recognition (CVPR 2004), Washington, USA, pp. 790–797 (2004)
11. Dame, A., Marchand, E.: Accurate real-time tracking using mutual information. In: Proceedings of the IEEE Int. Symp. on Mixed and Augmented Reality (ISMAR 2010), Taipei, Taiwan, pp. 47–56 (October 2010)
12. Pluim, J., Maintz, J.A., Viergever, M.: Mutual information based registration of medical images: a survey. Proceedings of IEEE Transactions on Medical Imaging 22(8), 986–1004 (2003)
13. Ramey, N.A., Corso, J.J., Lau, W.W., Burschka, D., Hager, G.D.: Real-time 3D Surface Tracking and Its Applications. In: Proceedings of IEEE Conference on Computer Vision and Pattern Recognition Workshop (CVPRW 2004), Washington, USA, pp. 33–34 (2004)

DOF Minimization for Optimized Shape Control under Active Constraints for a Hyper-redundant Flexible Robot

Valentina Vitiello, Ka-Wai Kwok, Christopher Payne, and Guang-Zhong Yang

The Hamlyn Centre for Robotic Surgery
Imperial College London, London, UK
{vvitiell,kkwok,christopher.payne04,g.z.yang}@imperial.ac.uk

Abstract. In robotic-assisted minimally invasive surgery, there are increasing interests in the use of articulated hyper-redundant robots to provide enhanced flexibility to conform to complex anatomical pathways without the constraint of accurate port placement. However, as the number of joints to be simultaneously actuated increases, so too does the complexity of the control architecture and the computational power required to integrate techniques such as adaptive force control and haptic feedback. In this paper, we propose a degree-of-freedom (DOF) minimization scheme for simplifying the control of a generic hyper-redundant articulated robot by identifying the minimum number of joints required to perform a specific task without compromising workspace limits. In particular, a time-varying instrument path is defined for realistic, *in vivo* settings involving tissue deformation. The minimum number of DOF is determined by the amount of angular displacement of the joints to ensure shape conformance and seamless trajectory manipulation. Dynamic active constraints are also imposed on the entire length of the flexible robot. Detailed simulation and preliminary experimental results are provided to demonstrate the practical application of the proposed framework.

Keywords: Medical Robotics, kinematic control, hyper-redundant robots, dynamic active constraints.

1 Introduction

In the past decades, Minimally Invasive Surgery (MIS) has brought extensive changes to the general practice of surgery. In spite of established benefits such as smaller incisions, reduced recovery time and minimal post-operative pain, the surgery itself presents many ergonomic and technical challenges due to instrument design and port access issues. The application of robotic technologies to MIS has significantly improved its functionality and usability through aligned visual-motor axes, 3D vision, motion scaling and intuitive instrument control [1]. In an attempt to overcome the limitations of the existing robotic surgical platforms, particularly for those related to rigid instrument design, current research is increasingly focused on the development of flexible instruments that enable more complex procedures to be performed [2]. The use of an articulated hyper-redundant robot allows increased flexibility since the body of the robot can follow complex trajectories. The use of a large number of joint units

R.H. Taylor and G.-Z. Yang (Eds.): IPCAI 2011, LNCS 6689, pp. 67–78, 2011.

also increases the fault tolerance of the robot. In addition, serial link mechanisms offer advantages such as the possibility of integrating inner channels to pass imaging probes, camera and other instruments. They also provide increased design flexibility, facilitate the integration of active constraints and help to maintain a desired shape thanks to the stiffness of the unactuated joints.

The problem of kinematic control for redundant manipulators has been extensively studied by the robotics community. In addition to the inverse kinematic method, which aims to find the joint displacements directly, Jacobian-based, gradient projection and task space augmentation approaches, which address the joint velocity solution, can be applied [3]. More recently, several authors have proposed the use of parametric curves to describe the geometric shape of redundant robots [4]. In spite of the theoretical validity of these simulation frameworks, which provide instantaneous solutions allowing for on-line path modifications, technical hurdles still prevent their application into physical realization. In particular, the simultaneous actuation of a large number of degrees of freedom (DOF) significantly increases both hardware and software control complexity. For MIS applications, this complexity is further enhanced if haptic guidance and active constraints are integrated for safer operation. In this paper, we propose a DOF optimization scheme that overcomes some of these difficulties by identifying the minimum number of active joints to be simultaneously actuated and constrained for a specific task. It can be used prior to surgery to estimate the desired motion of the joints and then be implemented together with sensing feedback to adapt to intra-operative changes. This simplifies the formulation of the kinematic solution whilst still addressing the motion of each individual joint. Another advantage of the proposed method over shape control algorithms is the use of a volumetric manipulation margin rather than a specific 3D parametric curve to be followed without any tolerance. This accounts for improved flexibility of manual control and its integration.

With the proposed method, a time-varying instrument path is defined along the surface of a deforming tissue model. The dynamic surgical model can be obtained by pre-operative imaging on a specific patient so that the shape of the instrument path can be registered with the super-imposed active constraint. A generic snake-like articulated robotic instrument is used. The method then utilizes an optimization algorithm to identify the optimum number of active DOF required to maintain dynamic shape conformance for the given surgical task. The kinematics of the robot can also be easily modified without affecting the algorithm, thus allowing its application to multiple robot configurations and surgical tasks. In this work, dynamic active constraints are imposed on the entire length of the robot body and detailed simulation results are used to assess the practical value of the technique. Furthermore, preliminary experimental validation is provided using a prototype articulated flexible access device to demonstrate its practical value.

2 Methodology

A dynamic surgical scene with a large amount of deformation is used for this study. The method is divided in two main steps: 1) determination of a set of optimal redundant configurations using an optimization algorithm; 2) minimization of the number of active DOF and application of the active constraint for validation.

2.1 Robot Configuration

For numerical assessment of the proposed algorithm, a generic 30-DOF snake-like robot is considered. It consists of 15 rigid links of equal length connected by universal joints. Each link is represented as a 20mm long cylinder and each universal joint as a sphere, both 10mm in diameter. Such modular structure simplifies the kinematic formulation for real-time control and practical applications. For kinematic analysis, a local coordinate system is defined for each link with the origin specified at the centre of the sphere representing the actuating universal joint. The origin of the world coordinate frame is instead placed at the origin of the active constraint model. The transformation between two consecutive link frames i and i+1 can be expressed in terms of the ith universal joint angles $q_{i,1}$, $q_{i,2}$ and the length of the link L as a 4x4 matrix T_i^{i+1}. The overall forward kinematic equations describing the position and orientation of the end-effector with respect to the world reference frame are therefore given by:

$$T_0^n(\mathbf{q}) = T_0^1 \prod_{i=1}^{n} T_i^{i+1}(q_{i,1}, q_{i,2}) \tag{1}$$

where n is the number of links, $\mathbf{q}=(q_{1,1},q_{1,2},\ldots,q_{i,1},q_{i,2},\ldots,q_{n,1},q_{n,2})$ is the vector of the joint variables and T_0^1 is the matrix defining the pose of the first link with respect to the world reference frame. It is important to note that this study only addresses the shape of the robot's body while the "head" is free to move outside the active constraint and can be directly controlled by the surgeon.

2.2 Surgical Scenario

The surgical scenario used for kinematic analysis in this study is laparoscopic liver resection. It is technically complex, involving a high risk of hemorrhage and gas embolism, and is hampered by the limitation of exploring the deeper regions of the organ. According to Couinaud's classification, only the anterolateral 2 to 6 Segments of the liver are considered consistent with the laparoscopic approach, while the upper right part of the organ (Segments 7 and 8) is difficult to reach with standard instrumentation (Fig. 1(a)). As shown in Fig.1(b), laparoscopic resection of lesions in the right side of the liver involves the use of 4 instrument ports on the patient abdomen [5]. In addition, both respiratory and cardiac cycles affect the shape of the liver generating large tissue deformation. The use of an articulated robotic instrument in such a scenario could improve the outcome of the procedure by ensuring safe navigation to the operative site and augmented stability for operation. The complexity of the instrument path together with the high amount of deformation makes this surgical scenario particularly challenging, and thus is ideal for assessing the validity of our method.

For the purpose of this study, a virtual lesion to be excised through a minimally invasive approach is located on the back surface of the liver at the level of Segment 7.

An example path to be followed by the flexible instrument is defined along the surface of the liver and a dynamic active constraint is superimposed delimiting the safe region of navigation, as shown in Fig. 2. To be consistent with the laparoscopic configuration, the first point of the path representing the entry point of the instrument on the patient's body is fixed and located in the lower-left part of the liver (Fig. 2, left). The last point is placed in correspondence of the liver lesion behind Segment 7 and is kept stationary to ensure adequate stability, since it determines the location of the head of the robot which is free to move for surgical operation and not shown in the model (Fig. 2, right).

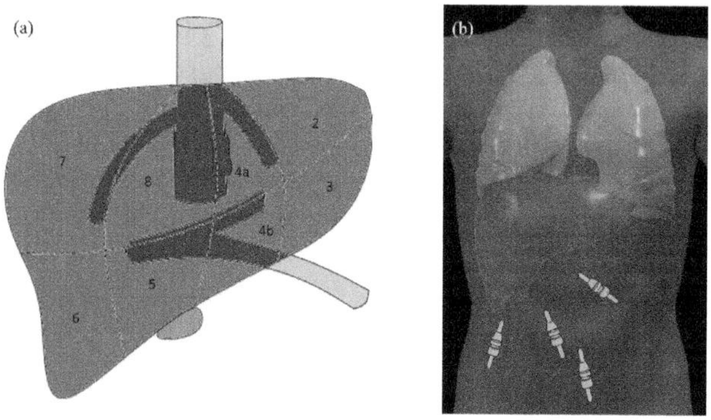

Fig. 1. Anatomical considerations for laparoscopic liver surgery. (a) Couinaud classification of liver's Segments; (b) Typical port placement for resection of lesions in segments 5 through 8.

2.3 Active Constraints

Safe manipulation of articulated robotic devices in MIS requires consideration of the allowable workspace coupled with the anatomical structures surrounding the entire body of the device, rather than simply the motion of a single-point end-effector. Relying on the buttressing of anatomical structures to constrain or guide the device is considered to be unsafe and insufficient for protecting the delicate tissues from being accidently perforated. In order to provide a safety boundary with explicit manipulation margins for the entire articulated device, we recently proposed a real-time modeling scheme [6] to construct a smooth cylindrical pathway with detailed geometric constraints. This follows the concept of dynamic active constraint/virtual fixtures, which can react and adapt to tissue deformation.

Pre-operatively, a surgical planning interface is provided to enable the operator to set a reference pathway defining a volumetric margin for the articulated robot. In order to avoid the defined pathway colliding with the anatomical models and to enable accurate prescription, a haptic device (Omni Phantom, Sensable Tech. Inc., USA) is used as a 3D coordinate input device to indicate contact with the anatomical models during the placement of the control points. The deforming 3D model of the liver used for this study is reconstructed by segmentation of pre-operative 4D CT scan images of a real patient. The maximum displacement of the diaphragm for this specific case is 16mm. The corresponding peak-to-peak maximum deformation of the

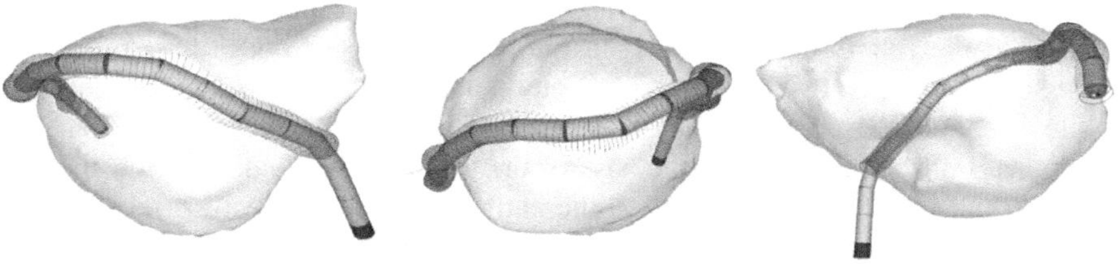

Fig. 2. Active constraint modeled on the surface of the liver from three different perspectives. The constraint dynamically adjusts its shape according to the liver deformation due to respiratory and cardiac cycles. The corresponding optimal configuration of the redundant snake-like robot inside the active constraint is also shown.

constraint adapting to the induced liver deformation is about 14.5mm. As previously explained, this model is used to predict the desired joint motion and has to be integrated with intra-operative data for *in vivo* applications. As an example, a real-time dynamic shape instantiation method has recently been developed to obtain a detailed 3D deformation model of the liver using imaging data [7]. Proximity query is performed offline to compute the deviation of the robot into the forbidden region defined as outside the volume prescribed by the active constraints as described in [8].

3 Optimization Algorithm

As previously stated, the head of the snake robot is not considered in the optimization algorithm since it is directly controlled by the surgeon and free to move outside the constraint. The optimal configuration at each time-frame is therefore determined by ensuring that the position of the end-effector remains stationary while the body of the robot conforms to the pre-defined trajectory. This condition can be fulfilled by constraining the motion of each link independently, thus eliminating the need of expressing the inverse kinematics of the end-effector in a closed-form solution. Such a task is highly computationally demanding for hyper-redundant mechanisms and involves the use of a pseudo-inverse Jacobian matrix, which causes stability issues when using velocity control [3].

3.1 Singularities and Local Minima

Two singularity conditions must be addressed to ensure the stability of kinematic control methods: position singularities and reduced-rank Jacobian singularities [3]. Reduced-rank Jacobian singularities are related to the dexterity of the robot's head, which is not involved in the optimization. Nonetheless, singularities can still occur when the trajectory between two consecutive timeframes cannot be followed continuously due to solutions with large joint angle differences. This can be avoided by exploiting the hyper-redundancy so that the motion is equally distributed among different joints. This is ensured by minimizing the total joint angle displacement between consecutive timeframes. Such constraint is also important for preventing the algorithm from falling into local optima resulting from the multiple inverse kinematics solutions of redundant structures [3].

A position singularity normally occurs when a point of the end-effector trajectory is outside the robot workspace [3]. In our case, the robot body must possess the necessary flexibility to conform to various configurations with adequate accuracy while keeping a fixed end-effector position. This requires the introduction of an additional translational DOF at the base of the robot, corresponding to the sliding of the first link inside the trocar port on the patient abdomen. However, this motion is used only to compensate for the difference in path length between timeframes by varying the position of the first robot link and is not considered in the optimization.

3.2 Objective Function

Since the end-effector is assumed to be target locked, the performance equation for the selection of the optimal inverse kinematics solution does not include a measure of manipulability. The workspace and dexterity of the articulated instrument depend on the head configuration, which is in turn dictated by the type of surgical procedure. On the other hand, the main performance measure is the distance D between the robot's body and the constraint's centerline. Also to be minimized is the joint angle displacement between two consecutive configurations R, so that the objective function at the kth timeframe is given by:

$$F_k = k_d \frac{D_k}{D_{MAX}} + k_r \frac{R_k}{R_{MAX}} \tag{2}$$

where k_d and k_r are weights determining the importance of each measure in the selection of the optimal solution. Each measure is also normalized with respect to the maximum allowable value. Particularly, the maximum allowable distance between the robot's body and the constraint's centerline D_{MAX} corresponds to the maximum radius of the active constraint, since it defines the safe region of motion. In contrast to [9] where the active constraint is treated as a constraint of the optimization, this formulation allows the robot to deviate from the pre-set constraint. This increases the flexibility of the proposed algorithm, as it accounts for modifications of the volumetric shape of the constraint according to intra-operative changes. The maximum allowable angle displacement R_{MAX} is instead given by the physical limits of the micro-motor used for actuation. The range of motion of each joint is set as -45° and +45°. This is also set as the boundary limit for the search of the optimal solution $[\mathbf{q}_{lb},\mathbf{q}_{ub}]$. In addition, the physical limit of robotic actuation is also addressed by bounding the joint velocities $\dot{\mathbf{q}}$ according to the maximum motor speed in the range $[\dot{\mathbf{q}}_{lb}, \dot{\mathbf{q}}_{ub}] = [-\mathbf{1},\mathbf{1}] \cdot \pi$ rad/s. Assuming a very short time interval Δt between frames, the velocity limit can be converted to an angular displacement range referring to the joint configuration $\mathbf{q}_{k\text{-}1}$ optimized at the previous frame k-1. Thus, the overall constraint is expressed as:

$$\begin{cases} \mathbf{q}_{lb} \le \mathbf{q}_k \le \mathbf{q}_{ub} \\ \left(\Delta t \cdot \dot{\mathbf{q}}_{lb} + \mathbf{q}_{k-1}\right) \le \mathbf{q}_k \le \left(\Delta t \cdot \dot{\mathbf{q}}_{ub} + \mathbf{q}_{k-1}\right) \end{cases} \tag{3}$$

All the values of the constant parameters in Eq. (2) are reported in Table 1, where the Δt is based on a typical respiration rate of 15 cycles per minute. This is reasonable since most of the liver deformation is generated by respiratory motion.

Table 1. Values of the parameters in the objective function

k_d	k_r	D_{MAX}	R_{MAX}	k	Δt	n	L
1	0.5	9.04mm	90°	25	0.16s	15	20mm

The distance D between the robot's body and the constraint's centerline at the kth timeframe is defined as:

$$D_k = \sum_{i=1}^{n} \left\| \hat{\mathbf{x}}_i - \mathbf{x}_{i,k} \right\| \tag{4}$$

where $\mathbf{x}_{i,k}$ is the desired position of the ith universal joint on the constraint's centerline at the kth timeframe and $\hat{\mathbf{x}}_i$ is the actual position of the ith universal joint given by the first 3 elements of the fourth column of the matrix:

$$T_0^i = T_0^1 \sum_{j=1}^{i-1} T_j^{j+1}\left(q_{j,1}, q_{j,2}\right) \tag{5}$$

which is derived from Eq. (1) when $n=i$. The first universal joint is not considered in the optimization since it is located outside the active constraint (see Fig. 2) and its position is pre-defined by the transformation matrix T_0^1 according to the desired trajectory using the additional translational degree of freedom.

The joint angle displacement R at the kth timeframe is defined as:

$$R_k = \sum_{i=1}^{N_{DOF}} \left| \Delta q_i \right| \tag{6}$$

where $N_{DOF}=2n$ is the number of degrees of freedom and $\Delta q_i=q_{i,k}-q_{i,k-1}$ is the change in joint angle q_i with respect to the previous timeframe.

3.3 Optimization Results

The optimization algorithm is implemented in *Matlab* using the embedded function *fmincon* to find the inverse kinematic solution $\mathbf{q}_k$ within the allowable joint motion range at each timeframe by minimizing the value of F_k subject to the non-linear equality constraint:

$$\left\| \hat{\mathbf{x}}_n - \mathbf{x}_n \right\| = 0 \tag{7}$$

where $\mathbf{x}_n$ is the fixed desired position of the end-effector on the constraint's centerline and $\hat{\mathbf{x}}_n$ is the actual position of the end-effector given by the 3D translation vector of the transformation matrix (1). This condition ensures that the position of the end-effector remains constant at each timeframe.

A video showing the result of the optimization is provided in the supplementary material. The body of the robot successfully conforms to the deforming active constraint during the whole respiratory cycle without exceeding the maximum motor speed. All the values of the simulation parameters are reported in Table 2. The maximum joint angular velocity $\dot{q}_{max}$ is found to be 1.5018 rad/s and the computational time t_{comp} is 336 s. This is reported as a measure of complexity to show how it decreases with the number of active DOF since the method is not supposed to be used real-time. The minimum value of the objective function is always below 0.3481 and the maximum deviation outside the safety region p_{max} is 1.4763 mm. This error occurs at the end of the path corresponding to a particularly tortuous and narrow section of the constraint, as visible in Fig. 2. The use of shorter rigid links would allow for more accurate shape matching in this region; however, the force exerted on the tissue resulting by such a small deviation should not generate safety issues.

Table 2. Values of the optimization parameters obtained in this study

N_{DOF}	t_{comp} [s]	$\bar{F}$	F_{max}	$\dot{q}_{max}$ [rad/s]	$\bar{p}$ [mm]	p_{max} [mm]
30	336	0.1048	0.3481	1.5018	0.0214	1.4763
7	42	1.1452	2.1245	1.4754	0.0422	2.2133
6	28	1.3947	2.3770	1.4962	0.0534	2.7968
5	26	1.7564	3.1930	1.4548	0.0665	3.2888
4	14	2.5600	4.6378	1.5439	0.0902	3.6481
3	6	4.8425	9.2502	1.5439	0.3912	8.3331

4 DOF Minimization

Once the optimal inverse kinematics solution is found, the amount of angular displacement for each joint among all timeframes is computed. The necessary DOF are then identified as the ones with a joint motion range higher than 0.2 rad. This value is chosen by comparing the average and maximum angular displacement. In this specific case, 7 DOF are needed to ensure shape conformance. The optimization algorithm is implemented again to compute the optimal inverse kinematics solution when only the selected joints are free to move and the others remain fixed. The optimal hyper-redundant solution corresponding to the 13th timeframe is chosen as the initial configuration since it features an average amount of deformation during the respiratory cycle and the result of the optimization largely depends on the values of the fixed joints. Once the minimum DOF configuration is determined, the number of active joints is further decreased by fixing one at a time the degree of freedom with minimum angular displacement over the different timeframes. The optimal inverse kinematics solution is determined in each case by using the proposed optimization algorithm and the corresponding results are reported in Table 2.

When the number of available degrees of freedom is decreased from 30 to 7, the computational time is reduced almost 10 times since the kinematics of the robot is much simpler, while the value of the maximum deviation is still approximitely 2 mm. Fig. 3 (left) shows the comparison of maximum deviation values at each time frame between three different cases: a fixed solution corresponding to the initial configuration, the minimized 7-DOF solution and the hyper-redundant solution. The periodic movement of the active constraint adapting to the liver deformation is clearly shown on the graph. Fig. 3 (left) also demonstrates that the maximum deviation is already more than halved by using only 7 DOF.

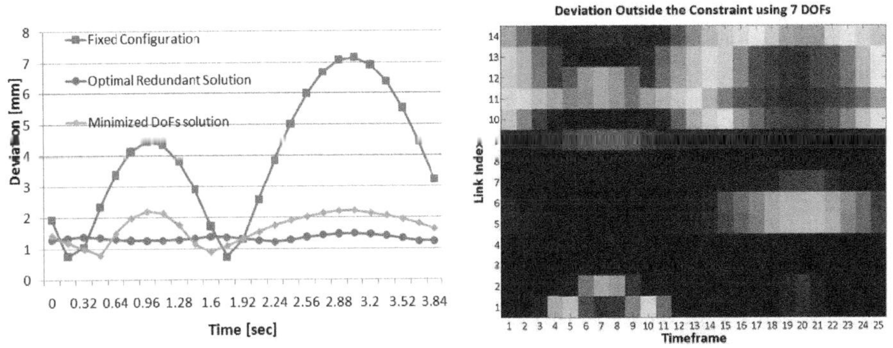

Fig. 3. Left: Comparison of maximum deviation values at each time frame between a fixed robot configuration (in blue), the 30-DOF (in red) and the minimized DOF (in green) solution; Right: Maximum deviation at each time frame for each link for the minimized DOF solution. Cold colors correspond to lower values of deviation.

It can be seen from Table 2 that the maximum deviation is less than 3 mm when using 6 DOF and below 4mm when using 5 or 4 DOF. Higher values of deviation are encountered when less DOF are used, which is as expected as the instrument now becomes more rigid. The maximum joint angular velocity is always lower than the motor speed limit and the mean value of the deviation $\overline{p}$ is much smaller than the maximum value. These results also suggest that when using a minimum number of DOF, only a small portion of the robot is beyond the active constraint. This is demonstrated in Fig. 3 (right), which shows that deviation mainly occurs in correspondence of the distal links.

5 Preliminary Experimental Validation

To demonstrate the practical application of the proposed algorithm, controlled laboratory experiments have been performed using an articulated flexible access device for MIS with embedded positional feedback. The robot is an early prototype of the 7-DOF system described in [10] featuring 5 independently controllable DOF arranged as two distal universal joints (intersecting pitch and yaw) and one proximal single DOF joint (yaw only). The angular displacement of each motor is sensed by a potentiometer mounted on the axis of rotation (see Fig. 4). The anatomical model is obtained by deforming a liver phantom with a custom mechanical device simulating the motion induced by the diaphragm during respiration. Optical markers are attached to the phantom to measure its deformation using an optical tracker (Optotrak Certus,

NDI, Canada) and reconstruct the surface to generate the active constraint (see Fig. 4). Details of the motion model and mechanical device can be found in [11].

The robot is mounted on an optical table and the active constraint in this case is imposed so that the first point and the overall path length are fixed during the motion. Also, due to the limited number of available DOF, the constraint on the fixed robot tip position is removed from both the active constraint and the optimization algorithm. The maximum displacement induced by the mechanical device on the liver phantom is 9.5mm and the corresponding peak-to-peak deformation of the constraint is 29mm. This high value is due to the fact that the phantom translation is not constrained in the laboratory environment. Fig. 4(a) shows the simulated robot and constraint configurations at the two extreme motion positions. The corresponding real robot configurations are depicted in Fig. 4(b) and (c).

To match the kinematic model of the robot with the one in Eq. (1), an additional constraint is introduced on the pitch axis of the proximal joint to keep its angular displacement equal to zero during the entire motion cycle. The three rigid links have equal length of 35mm plus 9mm of universal joint unit, giving a total of 44mm, while the diameter of the device is 12.5mm. Inverse kinematic control is implemented according to the angular values obtained from the optimization algorithm. Each cycle of the periodic motion has duration of 3sec and is divided in 23 equally spaced time frames selected from the tracking data.

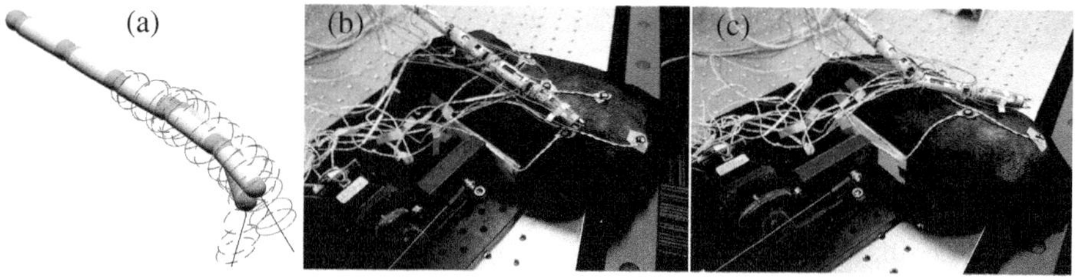

Fig. 4. (a) Configuration of the simulated robot inside the active constraint at the two extreme positions of full inspiration (blue dashed rings) and full expiration (red solid rings); Photos showing the articulated robot conforming to the surface of the liver phantom at two extreme configurations corresponding to full inspiration (b) and full expiration (c).

The graphs in Fig. 5 show the values of the potentiometer readings during one motion cycle with (b) and without (a) DOF minimization control. Motors are numbered incrementally from the most distal to the most proximal part of the robot. It is clear from the plot in Fig. 5(a) that motors 2 and 3 have the maximum angular displacement across all time frames, and therefore compensate for most of the deformation. The minimum number of DOF needed to ensure shape conformance in this case is only 2. Fig. 5(b) demonstrates that the control is able to keep motors 1, 4 and 5 at a fixed angular position in the 2-DOF case. The potentiometer readings are used in the simulation environment to compute again the forward kinematics of the robot (Eq. 1) and determine the maximum deviation outside the active constraint. The plot in Fig. 5(c) shows the corresponding value at each time frame for the 5-DOF and 2-DOF case. It is important to note that the deviation values are much lower with minimized DOF control. This is due to the fact that the simultaneous control and actuation of a higher number of DOF can be susceptible to errors and undesired jittery motion. These results demonstrate the practical application and validity of the proposed algorithm. It should be noted that the deformation of the liver can also be affected by interaction with the device itself or other instruments. Therefore, it is envisioned that the control architecture has to be refined by updating the inverse kinematic control in real-time on the basis of intraoperative imaging or sensing data. This can be implemented in a number of ways, such as Generalized Predictive Control or Kalman filtering.

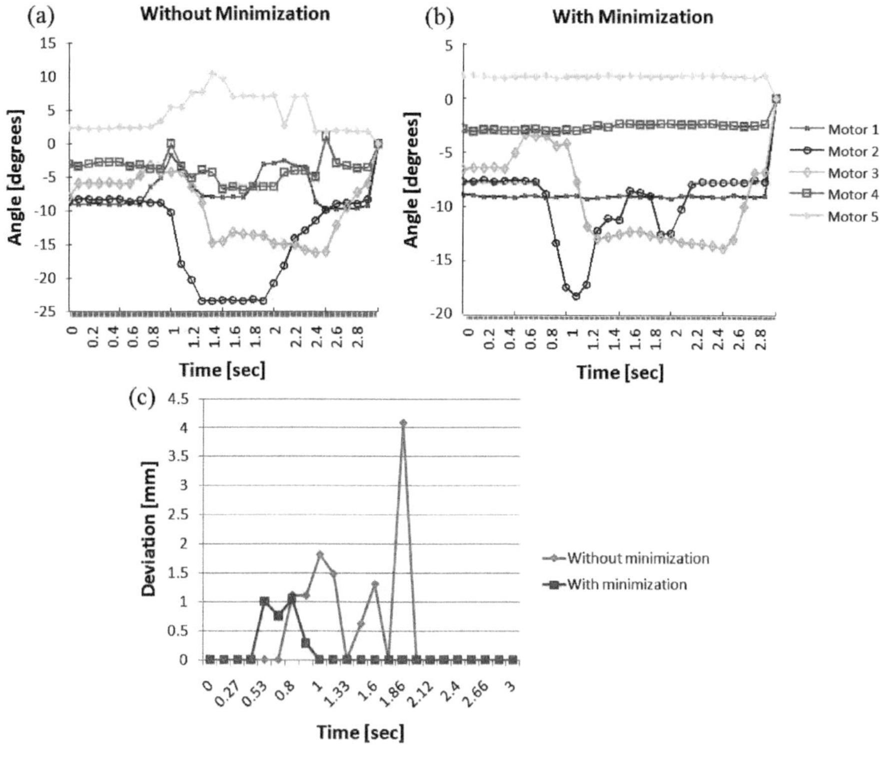

Fig. 5. (a) Plot of the potentiometer readings for the five simultaneously actuated motors during one cycle of motion; (b) Plot of the potentiometer readings for the five motors during one cycle of motion when only two DOF are used to ensure shape conformance while the rest are fixed; (c) Comparison of maximum deviation of the robot body from the constraint at each timeframe between the not minimized and minimized DOF case.

6 Conclusions

In this paper, we have proposed an effective method for optimizing the DOF of an articulated device for MIS to perform time-varying shape conforming tasks without entering a pre-defined forbidden region. Both simulation and preliminary laboratory results clearly demonstrate the practical value of the technique. The control principle is particularly relevant to the future implementation of robotic articulated instrument for NOTES such as the one used for preliminary experimental validation, for which path following and dynamic shape conformance are critical for its safe operation.

Acknowledgements. The authors wish to thank Dr. Jianzhong Shang and Mr. David Noonan for setting up the prototype articulated robot and Dr. Peter Mountney for assistance with the mechanical device and liver phantom used for validation.

References

1. Mack, M.J.: Minimally invasive and robotic surgery. J. Am. Med. Assoc. 285, 568–572 (2001)
2. Canes, D., Lehman, A.C., Farritor, S.M., Oleynikov, D., Desai, M.M.: The Future of NOTES Instrumentation: Flexible Robotics and In Vivo Minirobots. J. Endourol. 23, 787–792 (2009)
3. Siciliano, B.: Kinematic control of redundant robot manipulators: A tutorial. J. Intell. Robot. Syst. 3, 201–212 (1990)
4. Mochiyama, H., Shimemura, E., Kobayashi, H.: Shape Control of Manipulators with Hyper Degrees of Freedom. Int. J. Robot. Res. 18, 584–600 (1999)
5. Cho, J.Y., Han, H.-S., Yoon, Y.-S., Shin, S.-H.: Outcomes of laparoscopic liver resection for lesions located in the right side of the liver. Arch. Surg. 144, 25–29 (2009)
6. Kwok, K.-W., Mylonas, G.P., Sun, L.W., Lerotic, M., Clark, J., Athanasiou, T., Darzi, A., Yang, G.-Z.: Dynamic Active Constraints for Hyper-Redundant Flexible Robots. In: Yang, G.-Z., Hawkes, D., Rueckert, D., Noble, A., Taylor, C. (eds.) MICCAI 2009. LNCS, vol. 5761, pp. 410–417. Springer, Heidelberg (2009)
7. Lee, S.-L., Chung, A., Lerotic, M., Hawkins, M.A., Tait, D., Yang, G.-Z.: Dynamic Shape Instantiation for Intra-operative Guidance. In: Jiang, T., Navab, N., Pluim, J.P.W., Viergever, M.A. (eds.) MICCAI 2010. LNCS, vol. 6361, pp. 69–76. Springer, Heidelberg (2010)
8. Kwok, K.-W., Vitiello, V., Yang, G.-Z.: Control of Articulated Snake Robot under Dynamic Active Constraints. In: Jiang, T., Navab, N., Pluim, J.P.W., Viergever, M.A. (eds.) MICCAI 2010. LNCS, vol. 6363, pp. 229–236. Springer, Heidelberg (2010)
9. Kapoor, A., Li, M., Taylor, R.H.: Constrained control for surgical assistant robots. In: IEEE International Conference on Robotics and Automation, vol. 1, pp. 231–236. IEEE Press, New York (2006)
10. Shang, J., Noonan, D., Payne, C., Clark, J., Sodergren, M.H., Darzi, A., Yang, G.-Z.: An Articulated Universal Joint Based Flexible Access Robot for Minimally Invasive Surgery. In: IEEE International Conference on Robotics and Automation (accepted 2011)
11. Mountney, P., Yang, G.-Z.: Motion Compensated SLAM for Image Guided Surgery. In: Jiang, T., Navab, N., Pluim, J.P.W., Viergever, M.A. (eds.) MICCAI 2010. LNCS, vol. 6362, pp. 496–504. Springer, Heidelberg (2010)

A Robotic System for Intra-operative Trans-Rectal Ultrasound and Ultrasound Elastography in Radical Prostatectomy

Troy Adebar[1], Septimiu Salcudean[1], Sara Mahdavi[1], Mehdi Moradi[1], Christopher Nguan[2], and Larry Goldenberg[2]

[1] University of British Columbia, Vancouver BC V6T1Z4, Canada
[2] Vancouver General Hospital, Vancouver BC V6H0A5, Canada

Abstract. A new robotic system for trans-rectal ultrasound (TRUS) imaging during robot-assisted laparoscopic radical prostatectomy is described. The system consists of three main parts: a robotic probe manipulator (robot), an ultrasound machine with a biplane TRUS probe, and control and image processing software. A review of prior use of TRUS during prostatectomy is provided in order to demonstrate the potential benefits of such intra-operative imaging. The ability of the system to capture two-dimensional and three-dimensional B-mode and elastography data is demonstrated using a prostate phantom. A registration method that can be used for instrument tracking in RALRP is described and tested. Initial patient images captured using the system are presented.

Keywords: Image-guided surgery, robotic surgery, radical prostatectomy, trans-rectal ultrasound, medical image registration.

1 Introduction

Prostate cancer is the most commonly diagnosed cancer in North American men apart from skin cancer. In 2010, an estimated 24,600 new cases in Canada and 217,730 new cases in the United States will be diagnosed [2,1]. Common treatment options for prostate cancer include watchful waiting, radiation therapy and surgical intervention. Radical prostatectomy (RP), the surgical removal of the prostate gland and surrounding tissues, is viewed by many as the gold standard treatment for clinically-confined prostate cancer.

Several variants of RP exist: traditional open radical prostatectomy (ORP), laparoscopic radical prostatectomy (LRP), mini-laparotomy radical prostatectomy (MRP), and robot-assisted laparoscopic radical prostatectomy (RALRP) performed using the da Vinci Surgical System (Intuitive Surgical, Sunnyvale, CA). RALRP is quickly becoming the most popular variant with over 70 percent of procedures in the United States currently performed in this manner.

Radical prostatectomy is a technically challenging operation. A complete and accurate dissection is required to ensure removal of all cancerous tissue. Surgeons can experience difficulty in delineating the prostate boundary, in particular during dissection of the prostate apex and base. Surgeons must also tailor their

R.H. Taylor and G.-Z. Yang (Eds.): IPCAI 2011, LNCS 6689, pp. 79–89, 2011.

surgical margins to avoid the delicate nerves and blood vessels that form neurovascular bundles (NVB) around the periphery of the prostate. Damage to the NVB is thought to be a primary cause of post-operative impotence and incontinence, but the NVB are often extremely difficult to visualize due to their small size. Intra-operative imaging, in particular trans-rectal ultrasound, has the potential to reduce the challenges of RP by aiding surgeons in the delineation of critical periprostatic anatomy and the cancerous tissue.

This paper describes a new robotic system for intra-operative TRUS imaging in radical prostatectomy. Our system has two primary applications in RALRP. The first is capturing 3D ultrasound volumes of the prostate area immediately prior to surgery or during surgery for use in planning. Pre-operative surgical plans or pre-operative image data from MRI and other modalities can then be registered to the intra-operative ultrasound frame. This will allow surgeons to visualize the location of critical structures and patient-specific anatomy (e.g. accessory pudendal arteries). In the second application, surgeons will use real-time 2D TRUS imaging to visualize their surgical tools in relation to the periprostatic anatomy during surgery. Real-time B-mode, elastography and Doppler imaging will be available.

We will first review previous studies that have examined intra-operative TRUS in RP to motivate our work. We then describe our robotic TRUS system, as well as a method for ultrasound registration that can be used for automatic laparoscopic tool tracking in RALRP. Finally, we present imaging results from initial phantom and patient trials.

1.1 Review of Intra-operative TRUS in Prostatectomy

Intra-operative TRUS for guidance in prostatectomy was first reported in 1997 by Zisman et al. [14]. This group used TRUS in ORP during dissection of the prostate apex. Although their study was of limited size (n = 3), TRUS guidance was shown to be useful for identifying the boundaries of the prostate apex.

Several studies describing the use of TRUS in LRP have been published by Ukimura and Gill. Their first study described initial results using intra-operative B-mode, power Doppler and 3D TRUS imaging on twenty-five patients [11]. TRUS guidance was found to be particularly useful in identifying the correct plane between the bladder neck and the prostate base, identifying difficult-to-see distal protrusions of the prostate apex posterior to the membranous urethra, and providing visualization of any cancerous nodules abutting the prostate capsule, thus alerting the surgeon to perform a wider dissection at that point. Cancerous tissue was only vaguely visible in the B-mode images as hypoechoic regions. A detailed clinical study later found that TRUS significantly decreased the incidence of positive margins from 29 percent to 9 percent of patients [10].

A recent study investigated the effect of TRUS guidance on positive margin rates in mini-laparotomy prostatectomy (MRP), and used TRUS to measure the post-operative membranous urethral length (MUL) in order to examine its effect on post-operative continence [6]. TRUS was found to decrease distal positive margins from 23 percent to 12 percent of patients.

The first reported use of TRUS for guidance in RALRP was by van der Poel et al. in 2008 [8]. This group used TRUS to identify the correct plane between the bladder and the prostate base. The first 80 robotic operations by two experienced laparoscopic surgeons were compared. One surgeon used intra-operative TRUS, the other did not. In the first 30 cases, there was a significant difference in the rate of positive basal margins between the TRUS and non-TRUS surgeons. In the last 30 cases, there was no significant difference.

In a recent article, Han et al. describe a robotic TRUS probe manipulator to be used for guidance during RALRP [3]. This robotic manipulator overcomes the main limitation of all the previous studies: the need for a dedicated ultrasound assistant. In RALRP in particular, the da Vinci robot limits the assistant's access to the patient. Han et al.'s system allows the surgeon to reposition the probe directly using a computer joystick. Their system also allows for 3D reconstruction of ultrasound images using the TRUS robot's kinematics.

2 Materials and Method

2.1 Robotic TRUS Imaging System

Our robotic system for intra-operative TRUS imaging in prostatectomy consists of three main parts: a robotic probe manipulator (robot), an ultrasound machine with TRUS probe, and control and image processing software.

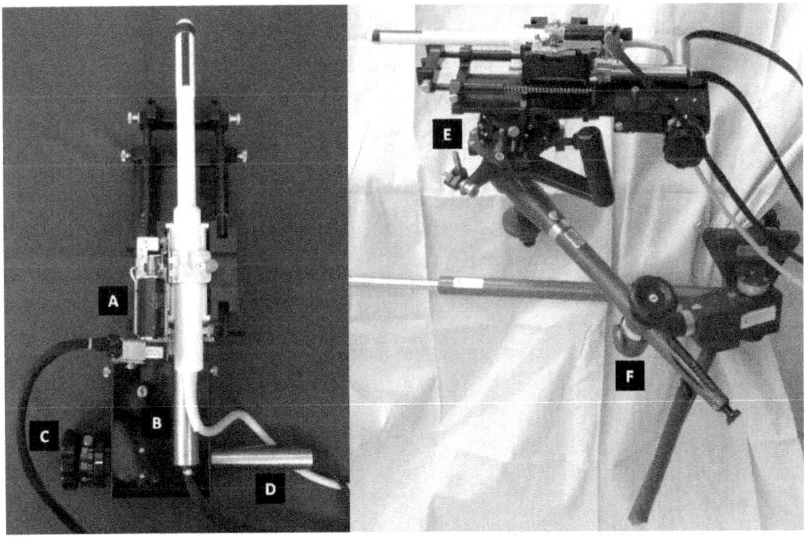

Fig. 1. Views of the robotic TRUS probe manipulator and stabilizer arm showing: (A) vibration assembly (B) roll motor (C) manual translation drum (D) translation motor (E) stabilizer fine adjustment stage (F) stabilizer gross adjustment clamp

The robot, shown in Figure 1, is based on a conventional brachytherapy stepper (EXII; CIVCO Medical Solutions, Kalona, IA), which allows the user to manually rotate the TRUS probe about its axis and manually translate (step) the TRUS probe along its axis. This particular stepper model originally had optical encoders attached to both movement assemblies that allowed the user to track the position of the TRUS probe using a reader. In our robot, the encoders have been replaced with servomotors that allow automatic rotation and translation of the probe. The probe holder section of the stepper has also been replaced with a module that can produce controlled radial vibration of the TRUS probe for ultrasound elastography imaging. The probe is held on a linear bearing while a servomotor spinning an eccentric cam vibrates the probe. The frequency of vibration is determined by the rotational speed of the motor shaft, while the amplitude of vibration can be adjusted mechanically. Robot motion parameters are listed in Table 1.

Table 1. Robot motion parameters

Parameter	Roll Stage	Translation Stage	Vibration Stage
Motor model	Faulhaber 2342	Faulhaber 2342	Maxon 11875
Gearmotor reduction	14:1	3.71:1	1:1
Motion range	±45 deg.	±60 mm	±2 mm
Response time (center to max)	1027 ms	905 ms	N/A
Resolution	3.5×10^{-3} deg.	5.3×10^{-3} mm	∞

A parasagittal/transverse biplane TRUS probe is used in combination with a PC-based ultrasound console (Sonix RP; Ultrasonix Medical Corp., Richmond, BC). Software running on the ultrasound console directs the robot movement and the ultrasound data acquisition. Currently, a simple graphical user interface (GUI) allows the user to position the probe, and automatically collect 2D B-mode images and radio-frequency (RF) data while rotating or translating.

Ultrasound elastography is a technique for measuring mechanical properties of tissue [7]. When compressed, softer tissue experiences larger strain than stiffer tissue. By vibrating the tissue and measuring the amount of tissue displacement or strain from consecutive RF-data images, characteristics such as elasticity or viscosity can be obtained. A variety of algorithms can be used to reconstruct the tissue properties, but a detailed description is outside the scope of this paper. In this work, we present only axial strain images. To capture elastography data using our system, the TRUS probe is vibrated by the mechanism described above during the acquisition of RF data. The vibration frequency content can be controlled by the user through the GUI. Image analysis software developed by our group [13] is used to generate 2D ultrasound elastography data either in real time or offline.

As with the system of Han et al., our system can be used to collect 3D data by translating or rotating the 2D imaging planes and automatically recording the encoder positions for each image. The 3D reconstruction takes place offline, and can be applied to either elastography or B-mode images.

2.2 Registration

We recently described a method for 3D ultrasound to stereoscopic camera registration through an air-tissue boundary [12] that can be used to register the TRUS images to the da Vinci camera. This registration method uses features pressed into an air-tissue boundary that can be imaged by 3D ultrasound through the tissue and by stereoscopic cameras through the air. Since these features can be identified in both frames, they can be used as common points for solving a rigid transformation between the camera and ultrasound coordinate frames. The registration error using this technique is significantly lower than obtained with previous methods based on external tracking systems. The robotic system described in this paper can be used in RALRP to capture the 3D ultrasound data needed for the registration. 2D or 3D TRUS images can then be overlaid in the correct orientation in the da Vinci operator's view.

This registration concept can also be applied to allow our robot to automatically track the da Vinci tool tips with the TRUS imaging planes, thus providing optimal guidance without any distraction to the surgeon. Tracking the tool tips with the ultrasound requires simply that the positions of the tool tips ${}^0x$ in the ultrasound frame $\{\underset{\sim}{o}_0, \underset{\sim}{C}_0\}$ be known in real time. The da Vinci API provides the location of the tool tips ${}^1x$ in the da Vinci frame $\{\underset{\sim}{o}_1, \underset{\sim}{C}_1\}$. Our registration method can be used to determine the transformation between the frames ${}^0T_1$. In this study we tested the accuracy of this registration for tracking. We simulated the da Vinci API by attaching optical markers to a da Vinci tool (Black Diamond Micro Forceps; Intuitive Surgical, Sunnyvale, CA) and tracking the tool tip using a Micron Tracker optical tracking system (H3-60; Claron Technology, Toronto, ON). The TRUS imaging frame was registered to the Micron Tracker frame through a PVC tissue phantom using a fiducial tool as previously described [12]. The da Vinci tool tip was then pressed against the surface of the phantom at multiple locations. At each location, the position of the tip in the Micron Tracker frame was recorded, and 2D B-mode ultrasound images with position data were recorded and processed into 3D volumes. The tool tip was manually localized in the resulting ultrasound volumes. The registration error was defined as the Euclidean distance between the ultrasound position and the registered Micron Tracker position. In essence, this error compares the ideal tracking location found manually in the ultrasound volume with the tracking location that was predicted by our registration method and the simulated da Vinci kinematics.

2.3 Ultrasound Data Acquisition Trials

Our system's various imaging modes have been tested in both *in vitro* and *in vivo* settings.

A specialized prostate elastography phantom (Model 066; CIRS, Norfolk, VA) was imaged. This phantom contains structures that simulate the prostate, urethra, seminal vesicles and rectal wall. The simulated prostate also contains three 1-cm diameter lesions which are designed to be invisible in B-mode images but visible in elastography images. Two-dimensional B-mode and axial strain elastography images of the prostate inclusions were captured in real time using both imaging arrays. B-mode and RF data with position information were also captured using both imaging arrays, and 3D B-mode and 3D elastography data were generated offline. The 3D data were visualized and manually segmented using Stradwin [9].

After obtaining informed consent, eight patients with a mean age of 61.4 ± 5.9 years were imaged using our TRUS system over a period of 8 months. Patients were imaged in the operating room immediately prior to RALRP, after sedation and positioning for surgery but before insufflation or the docking of the da Vinci system. A standard brachytherapy stabilizer arm (Micro-Touch 610-911; CIVCO Medical Solutions, Kalona, IA) was mounted to the operating table and the robot was installed on the stabilizer. The stabilizer's coarse and fine positioning mechanisms were used to position the probe relative to the patient. The surgeon then manually inserted the probe into the rectum, and positioned the probe for imaging. Three-dimensional B-mode and RF data were captured by rotating the parasagittal array only. The probe was removed from the patient, and the robot and stabilizer were uninstalled before the surgery commenced. Three-dimensional B-mode and elastography volumes were generated offline. The 3D data were again visualized and manually segmented using Stradwin.

3 Results

3.1 Registration

Table 2 shows measured registration errors. Four registrations were performed, with registration error measured at ten tool positions for each registration. The average error for all four registrations was 2.37 mm.

Table 2. Mean errors (n = 10) between tool tip location and predicted location based on registration. Errors are presented in the anatomical frame of the patient, along the superior-inferior (e_{S-I}), medial-lateral (e_{M-L}) and anterior-posterior (e_{A-P}) axes.

	e_{S-I} (mm)	e_{M-L} (mm)	e_{A-P} (mm)	e_{Total} (mm)
Registration 1	1.01 ± 0.74	0.48 ± 0.28	1.29 ± 1.21	1.99 ± 1.08
Registration 2	0.98 ± 0.51	0.42 ± 0.33	2.26 ± 1.39	2.66 ± 1.29
Registration 3	1.69 ± 1.03	0.43 ± 0.22	1.57 ± 0.89	2.47 ± 1.22
Registration 4	1.83 ± 1.15	0.73 ± 0.41	1.01 ± 0.65	2.38 ± 1.15
Average	1.38 ± 0.97	0.52 ± 0.34	1.53 ± 1.17	2.37 ± 1.15

3.2 Phantom Images

Figure 2 shows 2D axial strain elastography images and B-mode images of the prostate elastography phantom captured in real time. In the B-mode images, the prostate inclusions cannot be clearly identified. In the elastography images, the inclusions are visible as the low intensity areas (low strain) within the prostate.

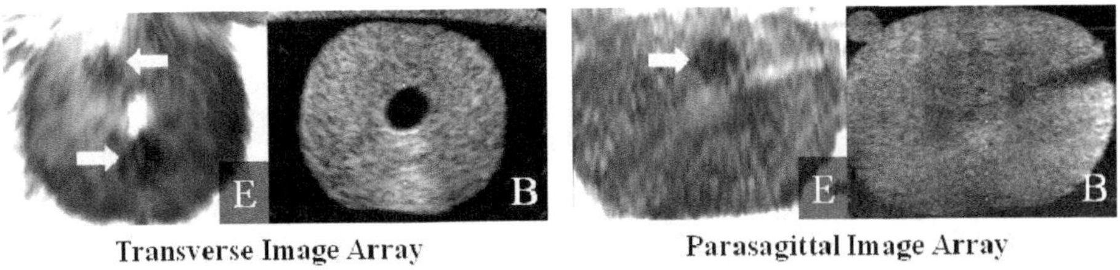

Fig. 2. Comparison of axial strain elastography (E) and B-mode images (B) of prostate elastography phantom. Arrows indicate inclusions in elastography images.

According to the phantom's documentation, the simulated lesions are approximately three times stiffer than the surrounding simulated prostate tissue. In the 8-bit (i.e. values from 0-255) strain images shown in Figure 2, the mean image intensity of the prostate excluding inclusions and urethra is 40.8 in the transverse image and 47.9 in the parasagittal image. The mean image intensity of the inclusions is 14.4 in the transverse image and 20.5 in the parasagittal image.

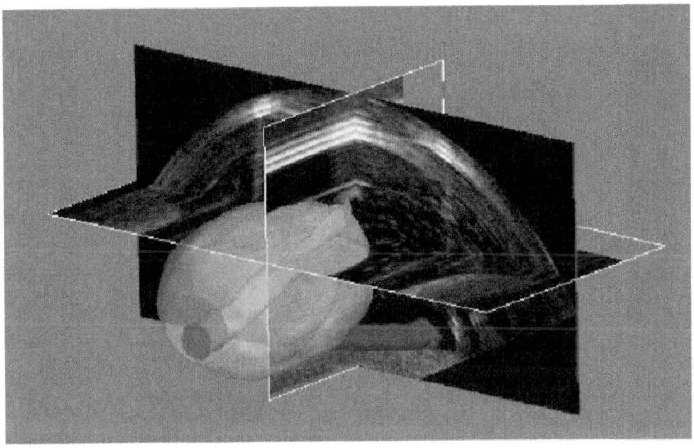

Fig. 3. Three-dimensional B-mode ultrasound of elastography phantom generated using the transverse imaging array.

Figure 3 shows a B-mode volume of the prostate elastography phantom captured by translating the transverse imaging plane. Orthogonal reslices of the volume data are shown, along with the manually segmented prostate, urethra and seminal vesicles.

3.3 Patient Images

Figure 4 shows axial strain elastography and B-mode patient images. The images shown are transverse-plane slices of the parasagittal volume data. The prostate boundaries are stronger in the elastography images than in the B-mode images.

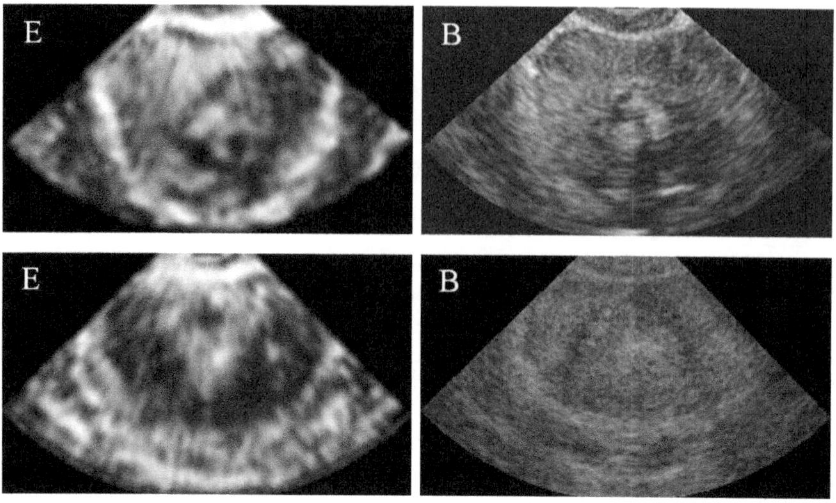

Fig. 4. Comparison of axial strain elastography (E) and B-mode images (B) of two patients

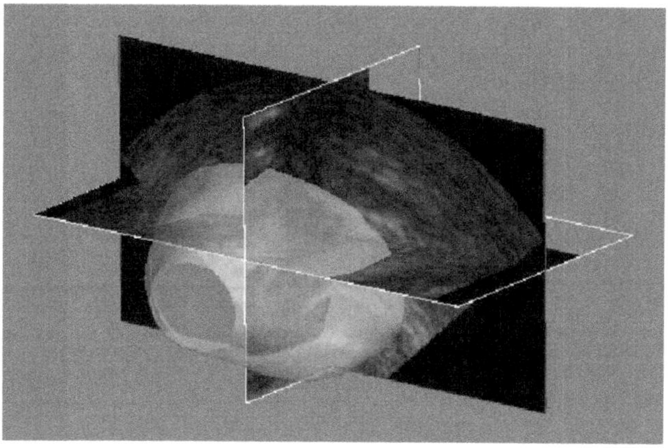

Fig. 5. Three-dimensional B-mode ultrasound of patient prostate generated using the sagittal imaging array

Figure 5 shows a B-mode volume generated from the patient data. Orthogonal reslices of the volume data are shown, along with the manually segmented prostate.

4 Discussion

Our TRUS system is well suited to intra-operative imaging in RALRP. The robot's large motion ranges (120 mm translation, 90 degrees rotation) allow even very large prostates to be imaged completely. Both the roll and translation stages have fast response times (both take approximately 1 second to move from zero position to maximum range). The robot and stabilizer arm do not interfere with the motion of the da Vinci arms, and because both are based on common clinical systems, they are straightforward for clinicians to install and position. Also, the system maintains the standard stepper's manual interfaces so that in the event of a failure or depending on their preference, the surgeon can elect to manipulate the device manually through all its degrees of freedom.

Automatic translation along the probe axis raises the issue of injury to the patient's rectum during probe movement. To address this concern, the translation motor is only slightly geared (3.71:1) so that the translation stage remains back-driveable. The force applied to the patient's rectum is restricted by hardware and software limits on the motor current, and both can be adjusted. All gross motions of the probe, including initial insertion, will continue to be performed manually by the surgeon. We plan to investigate the issue of force applied to the rectum in our future clinical work.

Compared to the system of Han et al., our system's primary advantages are its fully manual override and its ability to capture ultrasound elastography data. The phantom images shown in Figure 2 emphasize the advantage of ultrasound elastography imaging compared to B-mode imaging in prostatectomy. Although Ukimura and Gill have used B-mode ultrasound to identify cancerous tissue near the edge of the prostate [11], the specificity of B-mode ultrasound in prostate cancer detection is known to only be on the order of 50 percent. This means surgeons using B-mode images for guidance would not be able to reliably tailor their dissections according to intra-operative ultrasound. Our system's elastography capability will greatly improve the intra-operative visualization of cancerous tissue. Apart from cancer visualization, ultrasound elastography has also been shown to be more effective for imaging prostate anatomy in general than B-mode ultrasound [4], as seen in Figure 4 where the prostate boundaries are much clearer.

As discussed above, we foresee two usage modes for our system: 3D TRUS imaging for surgical planning and 2D TRUS imaging for real-time guidance. Both have some remaining technical challenges that will need to be overcome. The surgical planning use of the 3D images requires the registration of pre-operative MRI to intra-operative 3D ultrasound, a complex problem that has yet to be totally solved. We have previously reported rigid registration of MRI to TRUS elastography with reasonably small Dice similarity measures [5], but further work in this area, including non-rigid registration, will be needed. It may also be necessary to increase the speed of our 3D volume generation. Capturing 2D data with position information by rotating or translating the probe typically takes 60 to 90 seconds, although this can be adjusted by the user. Processing these data into a scan-converted volume takes approximately 280 seconds for B-mode data and between 8 and 15 minutes for elastography data depending on the reconstruction algorithm used. (Currently all 3D data is processed off-line.) It will likely be possible to optimize our processing in the future to near real-time performance, and certainly to a speed that will be practical for use in the OR. Finally, the real-time 2D image guidance use requires an interface for positioning the ultrasound plane that does not interrupt the surgeon's work flow. Automatic tool tracking using the registration method described above seems the best option. For a secondary, manual positioning option, we plan to move beyond our own simple GUI or the joystick control described by Han et al. to a more natural interface executed directly through the da Vinci console.

The overall average error previously reported for ultrasound to camera registration using our air-tissue boundary method was 1.69 ± 0.6 mm [12]. The overall average error in the current registration test was 2.37 ± 1.15 mm, 0.68 mm higher than the previous result. In that experiment, a cross-wire tool that could be tracked very accurately by the Micron Tracker was used to measure registration error. The increase in registration error in this experiment likely results from tracking the tip of the da Vinci forceps using the Micron Tracker. The Micron Tracker locates individual optical markers within 0.2 mm, but when it is used to track a tool tip with markers on the base, the error is exacerbated by a lever-arm effect. Based on the geometry of our markers and the forceps, the additional tool tip tracking error would be as high as 0.8 mm.

Even a true tracking error as high as 2-3 mm would likely still be acceptable. Since the goal of tracking is simply to have the tool tips appear in the TRUS images, errors in the axial and lateral ultrasound directions are irrelevant as long as the tool tips are within the image boundaries. And because the thickness of the TRUS beam at the anterior surface of the prostate is on the order of millimeters, small errors in the elevational direction likely are not critical.

5 Conclusion

The initial phantom and patient studies we have described have demonstrated the suitability of our new robotic system for intra-operative trans-rectal ultrasound in robot-assisted radical prostatectomy. Future work will examine the use of the system in surgery and determine the value that is added to the RALRP procedure.

Acknowledgments. This work was supported by NSERC and the Institute for Computing, Information and Cognitive Systems (ICICS) at UBC.

References

1. American Cancer Society: Cancer Facts and Figures 2010. Tech. rep., American Cancer Society, Atlanta (2010)
2. Canadian Cancer Society's Steering Committee: Canadian Cancer Statistics 2010. Tech. rep., Canadian Cancer Society, Toronto (2010)
3. Han, M., Kim, C., Mozer, P., Schäfer, F., Badaan, S., Vigaru, B., Tseng, K., Petrisor, D., Trock, B., Stoianovici, D.: Tandem-robot assisted laparoscopic radical prostatectomy to improve the neurovascular bundle visualization: A feasibility study. Urology 77(2), 502–506 (2011)

4. Mahdavi, S.S., Moradi, M., Wen, X., Morris, W.J., Salcudean, S.E.: Vibro-elastography for visualization of the prostate region: Method evaluation. In: Yang, G.-Z., Hawkes, D., Rueckert, D., Noble, A., Taylor, C. (eds.) MICCAI 2009. LNCS, vol. 5762, pp. 339–347. Springer, Heidelberg (2009)
5. Mahdavi, S.S., Morris, W.J., Spadinger, I., Chng, N., Goksel, O., Salcudean, S.E.: 3D Prostate Segmentation in Ultrasound Images Based on Tapered and Deformed Ellipsoids. In: Yang, G.-Z., Hawkes, D., Rueckert, D., Noble, A., Taylor, C. (eds.) MICCAI 2009. LNCS, vol. 5762, pp. 960–967. Springer, Heidelberg (2009)
6. Okihara, K., Kamoi, K., Kanazawa, M., Yamada, T., Ukimura, O., Kawauchi, A., Miki, T.: Transrectal ultrasound navigation during minilaparotomy retropubic radical prostatectomy: Impact on positive margin rates and prediction of earlier return to urinary continence. Int. J. Urol. 16(10), 820–825 (2009)
7. Ophir, J., Cespedes, I., Ponnekanti, H., Yazdi, Y., Li, X.: Elastography: a quantitative method for imaging the elasticity of biological tissues. Ultrasonic Imaging 13(2), 111–134 (1991)
8. van der Poel, H.G., de Blok, W., Bex, A., Meinhardt, W., Horenblas, S.: Peroperative transrectal ultrasonography-guided bladder neck dissection eases the learning of robot-assisted laparoscopic prostatectomy. BJU Int. 102(7), 849–852 (2008)
9. Treece, G.M., Prager, R.W., Gee, A.H.: Regularised marching tetrahedra: improved iso-surface extraction. Computers and Graphics 23(4), 583–598 (1999)
10. Ukimura, O., Gill, I.S.: Real-time transrectal ultrasound guidance during nerve sparing laparoscopic radical prostatectomy: pictorial essay. J. Urol. 175(4), 1311–1319 (2006)
11. Ukimura, O., Gill, I., Desai, M., Steinberg, A., Kilciler, M., Ng, C., Abreu, S., Spaliviero, M., Ramani, A., Kaouk, J., et al.: Real-time transrectal ultrasonography during laparoscopic radical prostatectomy. J. Urol. 172(1), 112–118 (2004)
12. Yip, M.C., Adebar, T.K., Rohling, R.N., Salcudean, S.E., Nguan, C.Y.: 3D Ultrasound to Stereoscopic Camera Registration through an Air-Tissue Boundary. In: Jiang, T., Navab, N., Pluim, J.P.W., Viergever, M.A. (eds.) MICCAI 2010. LNCS, vol. 6362, pp. 626–634. Springer, Heidelberg (2010)
13. Zahiri-Azar, R., Salcudean, S.E.: Motion estimation in ultrasound images using time domain cross correlation with prior estimates. IEEE Transactions on Biomedical Engineering 53(10), 1990–2000 (2006)
14. Zisman, A., Strauss, S., Siegel, Y.I., Manor, H., Lindner, A.: Transrectal ultrasonographically assisted radical retropubic prostatectomy. J. Ultrasound in Med. 16(12), 777 (1997)

Hand-Held Force Magnifier for Surgical Instruments

George Stetten[1,3,4], Bing Wu[2], Roberta Klatzky[2], John Galeotti[3], Mel Siegel[3], Randy Lee[4], Francis Mah[5], Andrew Eller[5], Joel Schuman[5], and Ralph Hollis[3]

[1] Department of Bioengineering, University of Pittsburgh
[2] Department of Psychology, Carnegie Mellon University
[3] Robotics Institute, Carnegie Mellon University
[4] Department of Biomedical Engineering, Carnegie Mellon University
[5] Department of Ophthalmology, University of Pittsburgh School of Medicine
http://www.vialab.org

Abstract. We present a novel and relatively simple method for magnifying forces perceived by an operator using a tool. A sensor measures the force between the tip of a tool and its handle held by the operator's fingers. These measurements are used to create a proportionally greater force between the handle and a brace attached to the operator's hand, providing an enhanced perception of forces between the tip of the tool and a target. We have designed and tested a prototype that is completely hand-held and thus can be easily manipulated to a wide variety of locations and orientations. Preliminary psychophysical evaluation demonstrates that the device improves the ability to detect and differentiate between small forces at the tip of the tool. Magnifying forces in this manner may provide an improved ability to perform delicate surgical procedures, while preserving the flexibility of a hand-held instrument.

Keywords: haptics, touch, robotic surgery, microsurgery, force magnifier, force-reflecting, steady hand.

1 Introduction

A need exists for improvement in the perception of forces by the sense of touch when using tools to perform delicate procedures. This is especially crucial in microsurgery. For example, surgeons routinely repair tiny blood vessels under a microscope that are far too delicate to be felt by the hand of the surgeon. Another key area for potential applications is ophthalmological surgery, in which we have recently been exploring techniques for image-guided intervention using optical coherence tomography [1]. Providing a useful sense of touch for such applications would improve outcome and increase safety.

Purely telerobotic systems such as the da Vinci® Surgical System (Intuitive Surgical, Inc., Sunnyvale, CA) can provide motion-scaling, so that fine motion of the tool can be controlled by coarser motion of the operator's hand on the controls. Although force at the tool tip cannot be sensed by the operator in the current commercial da Vinci® device, experimental systems have been tested that translate these forces into visual cues [2] as well as into vibrotactile feedback to the operators fingers [3].

R.H. Taylor and G.-Z. Yang (Eds.): IPCAI 2011, LNCS 6689, pp. 90–100, 2011.

A different, non-"tele"surgical approach has been demonstrated in several experimental systems, including the Force-Reflecting Motion-Scaling System created by Salcudean, et al. [4] [5], and the Steady Hand Robot described by Taylor, et al. [6][7]. These generate a magnified sense of touch by using a robotic arm that holds the surgical tool simultaneously with the surgeon, pushing and pulling as appropriate, to amplify the forces detected by small sensors between the handle of the tool and its tip. Because every force needs an opposing force, the robotic arm must be mounted somewhere, and being fairly massive, its weight must be supported by that mounting. Thus the magnified forces are created in these systems between the tool handle and subsequently the floor. To permit free motion of the tool by the surgeon, an elaborate remote-center-of-motion articulated robot arm is required, along with a control system to keep the tool moving naturally, as if controlled just by the operator, so that the surgeon can have something approaching the degrees of freedom and ease of manipulation that he/she is accustomed to with a freely held tool. Such systems are typically fairly extensive and complex. Issues involving the limited and congested workspace common in microsurgery raise serious challenges to practical deployment.

The desire to free robotic surgery devices from the floor-standing robotic arm has led to hand-held systems such as the Micron microsurgical instrument from Riviere's group, which uses piezoelectric actuators to move the tip relative to the handle, based on optical tracking of both the tip and handle [8]. The primary goal of Micron is to reduce the effects of hand tremor; it is not suited to provide a magnified sense of touch.

When the goal is to create additional forces for the operator to feel, some external frame to "push against" has generally been required. The field of haptic simulation faces the same dilemma of generating forces for the fingers to feel without anchoring the renderer to some solid base. Recent examples of more portable solutions include the "active thimble" described by Solazzi, et al. [9]. The device is entirely mounted on one hand. It attaches to the proximal part of the finger and reaches over to contact the fingertip, thus generating forces between two parts of the operator's own anatomy. As they describe it, "[a] limit of traditional kinesthetic interfaces is the difficulty to achieve a large workspace without a detriment of dynamic performance and transparency or without increasing the mechanical complexity. A possible solution to overcome this problem is to develop portable ungrounded devices that can display forces to the user hands or fingers."

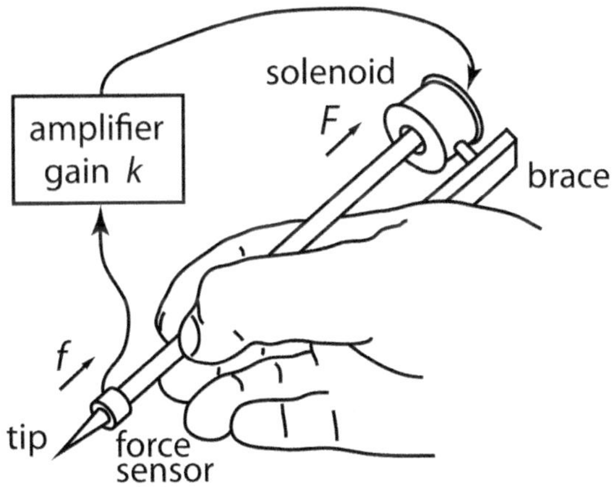

Fig. 1. The Hand-Held Force Magnifier (HHFM) uses a sensor to measure force f between the handle and the tip, which is amplified to produce a force $F = k f$ in the same direction on the handle using a solenoid mounted on the back of the hand.

In this paper we extend the concept of ungrounded haptic devices from purely virtual environments to real tools, by including a force sensor for interaction with an actual target. As in the Force-Reflecting and Steady Hand systems described above, we provide a magnified perception via the tool handle of forces sensed at the tool tip. Our device, however, does not require any freestanding apparatus, and instead produces forces between portions of the operator's own anatomy. The concept is shown in Fig. 1. A hand-held tool contains a sensor, which measures force f between the handle and the tip. This signal is amplified to produce a force F in the same direction on the handle of the tool using a solenoid mounted on the back of the hand. The human is, in effect, providing the moving platform from which the magnified forces are generated.

2 Design and Operation of the Device

Our Model-1 prototype of the Hand-Held Force Magnifier (HHFM) is illustrated in Fig. 2. In this first version, the tool tip is the small button on a force sensor (Honeywell FS01, 0-6.7 N). The tool handle is the body of a syringe attached to a piece of 1/4 inch brass tubing containing a stack of 8 permanent rare-earth magnets (3/16" Radio Shack 64-1895) inserted into a custom solenoid (250 ft of 30 gauge wire, 25 ohms, approx. 2360 turns). Magnets are used rather than simply a ferromagnetic plunger, so that forces can be generated in both directions. The solenoid is attached by a dual gimbal to a brace, which is mounted to the back of a wrist splint strapped to the operator's right hand. The dual gimbal decreases friction within the solenoid and increases flexibility of use by permitting free rotation in azimuth and altitude, while maintaining a tight connection for force in the range direction. A control system (not shown) includes a push-pull linear amplifier capable of supplying 32 V at 2 A, more than enough current to operate the solenoid over that voltage range. It employs simple proportional gain and permits adjustment of the offset to zero, to produce a force F from the solenoid of up to 1 N, proportional to, and in the same direction as, the force f sensed at the tool tip (Figs. 1 and 2). Thus we can express the system's behavior as simply

$$F = kf. \tag{1}$$

The proportionality factor k is adjustable from 0 to 5.8 in the Model-1. Above this level, the system becomes unstable, oscillating at approximately 400 Hz. Particular values of k (such as k = 2.4 used in the experiments described below) can be determined by linearly fitting known forces imposed at the sensor to corresponding generated forces measured at the solenoid (see Fig. 5). The value of k assumes that the plunger of the solenoid is in a fully extended state, which the operator is instructed to accomplish during normal operation by lightly pushing the tool handle forward before contacting a target. Higher values of k result if the plunger is pulled within the solenoid, as this results in stronger attraction between the coil and the permanent magnets for a given current.

The Model-1 prototype in Fig. 2 is shown being used to push a spring from the side to bend it. With the gain k set to 0, the spring is felt through the tool to be subjectively quite easy to bend. With k increased to maximum, the spring feels much harder to

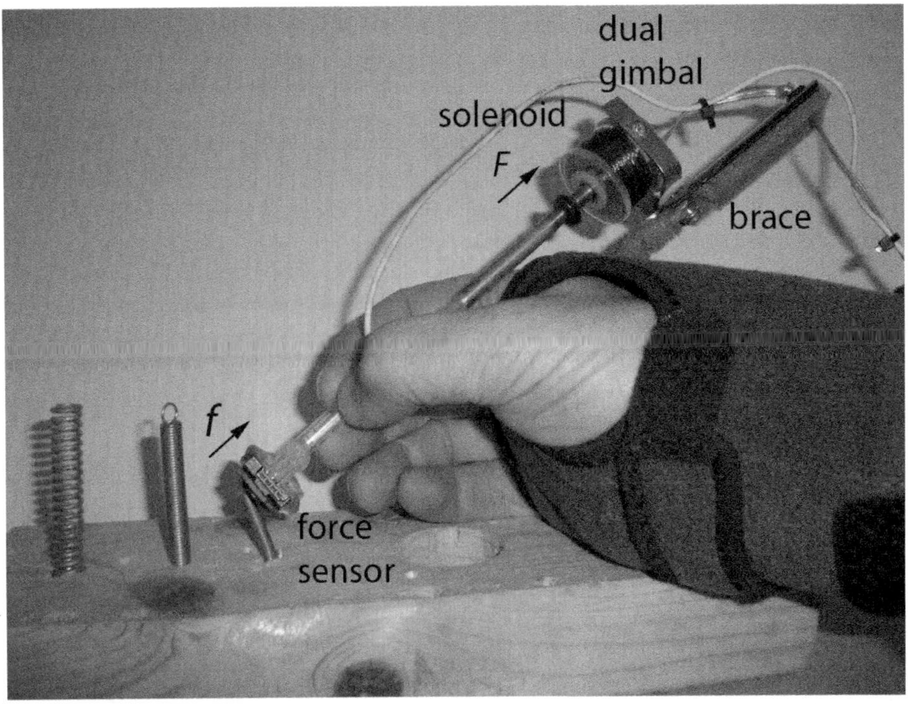

Fig. 2. Model-1 prototype of the Hand-Held Force Magnifier (HHFM). Here the operator "feels" a magnified version of the force generated by bending a spring.

bend. This haptic illusion is due to the fact that the fingertips must match not only the force of the spring *f* but also of that of the solenoid *F*. Thus the device magnifies the operator's sensation of touch. We hypothesize that the operator can sense forces at the tool tip that are smaller than would otherwise be perceivable, and can control these smaller forces with greater delicacy by interacting with the magnified forces. We report on preliminary tests of this hypothesis in the following section.

3 Psychophysics Experiments

Two experiments were conducted to characterize the Hand-Held Force Multiplier (HHFM). In the first experiment, the participants' ability to sense the presence of a force (i.e. the force detection threshold) was measured with and without the use of the HHFM. In the second experiment, we used a method of magnitude estimation to characterize the impact of the device on the subjective force intensity. Both studies produced a measure of the perceptual magnification of force implemented by the HHFM.

Experimental setup: The experimental setup (Fig. 3) consisted of a magnetic levitation haptic device (MLHD) from Butterfly Haptics (Maglev 200^{TM}, see http://butterflyhaptics.com) for rendering forces, a client computer for controlling stimuli and acquiring data, and a keypad for the participant to input responses.

The MLHD uses Lorentz forces for actuation, which arise from the electromagnetic interaction between current-carrying coils and magnets [10]. Since there are no motors, gears, bearings, or linkages present, it is free of static friction and able to generate forces precisely with a resolution of 0.02 N. In the present study, the MLHD was connected to a client PC through a 100 Mbps Ethernet cable. A multi-threaded application was run to command the MLHD to produce the desired stimuli and track the participant's responses from the keypad. Here the experimental stimuli were upward (counter-gravitational) forces ranging from 0.0-1.5 N. The forces were applied to the subject's hand while he or she held the HHFM (Fig. 3a) or an unmodified syringe (control condition) of the same diameter (Fig. 3b) in contact with the handle of the MLHD. The updating rate for force rendering was 2 kHz.

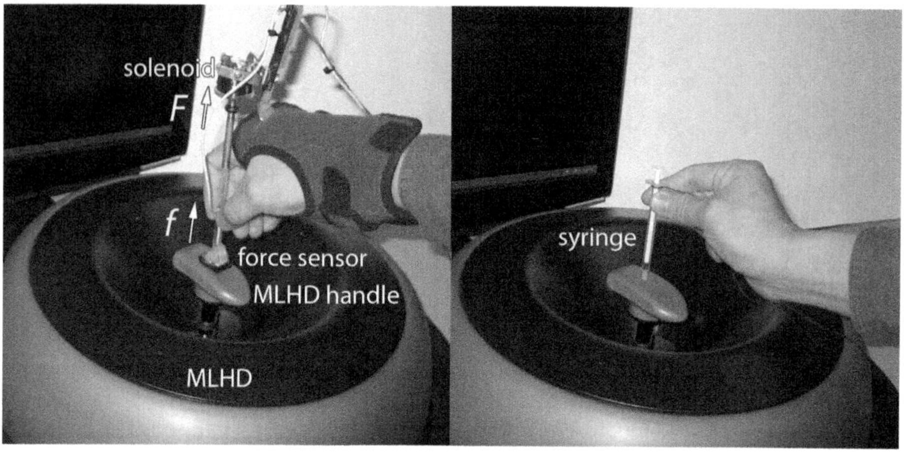

Fig. 3. Experimental setup for testing the Hand-Held Force Magnifier (HHFM). The user's perception of force was compared across the HHFM-on/off conditions (a) and control condition (b). A Magnetic Levitation Haptic Device (MLHD) was used to produce the experimental stimuli.

Experimental design: Participants were tested in three conditions in both experiments. In the HHFM-on and HHFM-off conditions, the participant put the device in his or her right hand and held the tubular portion between the thumb and index finger, as shown in Fig. 3a. He or she was instructed to hold the HHFM vertically, use it to press the MLHD handle, and so feel the vertical resisting force. Trials with the HHFM on or off were intermixed, and the experimenter controlled the state of the device with a switch as signaled by the computer without informing the participant. In the control condition (Fig. 3b), the participant held an unmodified syringe in the same way as the HHFM was held in the experimental conditions and felt the stimulus force transmitted through it.

Experiment 1: Force detection with the HHFM. Six participants, four males and two females, aged between 22 and 35, participated in this experiment with informed consent. All were right-handed by self-report and naïve to the purposes of this study.

Participants were tested individually with eyes closed. Each sat in a chair in front of the MLHD and adjusted the chair height to allow his or her right forearm to rest on the MLHD's top rim in a comfortable position. Active noise- cancelling headphones were worn to mask the sound from the environment. The participant was asked to hold the HHFM or the syringe and use it to touch the MLHD handle. A series of forces was then presented. In descending or ascending series, respectively, the initial force was clearly above (0.3-0.4 N) or below (0.0 N) the threshold, and thereafter the participant adjusted the force by pressing the "–" or "+" button until he or she felt that the stimulus had just disappeared or appeared. This procedure was repeated twice for each series. The threshold was then calculated as the mean value of the four threshold values.

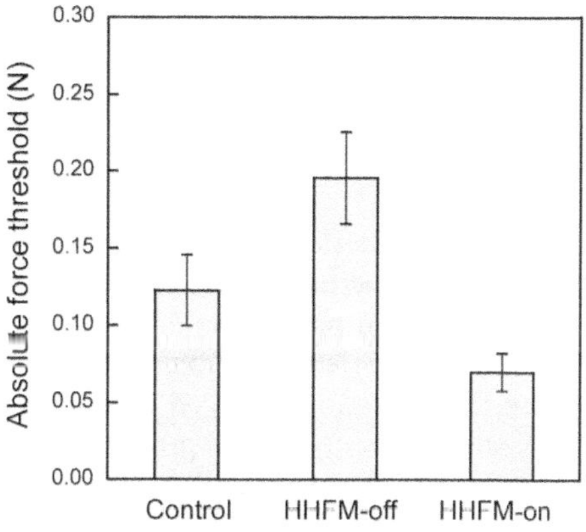

Fig. 4. Measured force detection thresholds. Error bars represent the standard error of the mean

Participants were tested first in the control condition and then in the HHFM on/off conditions. The testing order of HHFM-on and HHFM-off conditions was counterbalanced across participants.

Figure 4 plots the mean detection thresholds as a function of the experimental conditions. The mean threshold across all participants was 0.07 N in the HHFM-on condition, significantly lower than the threshold of 0.19N when the HHFM was off ($t(5)=3.99$, $p= 0.005$, one tailed paired t-test). The threshold of 0.12 N obtained in the control condition was significantly less than the HHFM-off condition, ($t(5)=5.85$, $p= 0.001$), possibly because of the additional weight of the device. Thus comparisons between the HHFM-on and control may be contaminated by weight, but a marginal advantage for HHFM-on relative to control was still found, ($t(5)=2.01$, $p= 0.05$).

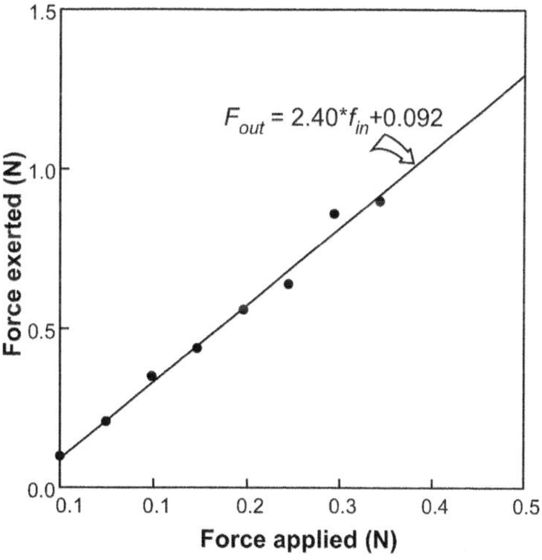

Fig. 5. Measured magnification factor k of the HHFM represented as the slope of a linear fit to a series of force measurements at the sensor compared to those at the solenoid

To quantify the perceptual magnification of the device, a measure was calculated as the ratio between the thresholds observed in the HHFM-on and HHFM-off conditions. Individual participants' perceived magnification yielded a confidence interval of 3.1 ± 1.2. This range includes the HHFMs actual total magnification, which we define to be $k + 1$, or 3.4, since the total force felt at the handle is $F + f$ (namely, the force from the solenoid plus that from the tip) and the value of k was determined to be 2.4 (see Fig. 5).

Experiment 2: Force estimation with the HHFM. The same six participants took part in this experiment. The experimental setup was the same as previously. A magnitude estimation procedure [11] was used, by which the participants freely assigned numbers (integers or fractions) to force stimuli, in relation to their perceived intensity. Each force was to be judged in isolation, with the only restriction being that greater subjective intensity should produce a greater numerical value.

The force stimuli were 0.1, 0.2, 0.3, & 0.4N. In addition, the forces of 0.5, 1.0, & 1.5N were used in the control trials to produce a similar response range for both control and HHFM trials and thus reduce possible range effects resulting from the HHFM magnification. Each force was tested three times in each condition. The three repetitions occurred in different blocks in random order, with a 5-minute break between blocks. As before, the HHFM-on and HHFM-off trials were intermixed so that the participants had no knowledge of the status of the HHFM. The order of control and HHFM conditions was counter-balanced across subjects. The entire experiment lasted approximately one hour.

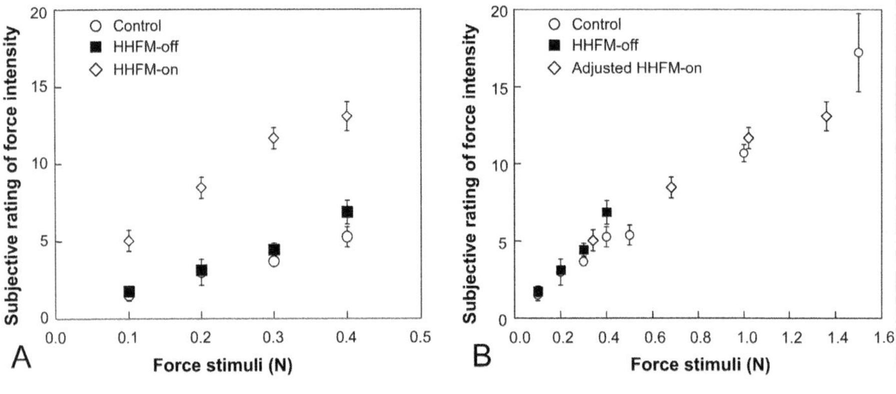

Fig. 6. (A) Mean judged magnitude for the stimulus forces. Error bars represent the standard error of the mean. (B) Plot of all data points, including the forces tested only in the control trials. Here the HHFM-on data were re-plotted versus the predicted output of the HHFM.

The data were normalized by dividing each judgment by the participant's mean within a given condition, and then multiplying by the grand mean for all participants. The three estimates from repeated measurements were averaged and taken as the estimated magnitude for each stimulus in each condition. Fig 6A shows the mean estimated magnitude, averaged across six subjects, for the forces tested in the three conditions. Perceptual magnification was then estimated for each participant as the slope of a linear regression relating the mean HHFM-on magnitude to the HHFM-off magnitude for each stimulus. The participants' perceived magnification ranged from 1.85 to 2.40 with a mean of 2.14 ± 0.18, somewhat less than the HHFM's total magnification factor determined above to be 3.4. If the HHFM-on curve was rescaled by multiplying each objective stimulus value (x-axis point) by the total magnification factor, as shown in Fig 6B, it essentially coincided with the curve obtained in the control condition.

Three two-way (force × device) repeated-measure ANOVAs were performed on the raw data to assess the effects of the HHFM on perceived force magnitude. The comparison of the HHFM-off and control data found only a significant main effect for force ($F(3,15)=16.61$, $p<0.001$), but showed no device effects ($F(1,5)=0.18$, $p=0.69$) or significant interaction ($F(3,15)=0.67$, $p=0.59$). That is, the additional weight of the HHFM did not affect subjective magnitude in this supra-threshold task, as it did the threshold in the previous experiment. The same ANOVA comparing HHFM-on to control showed, in contrast, higher magnitudes for the HHFM-on ($F(1,5)=20.76$, $p=0.006$) and a significant force × device interaction ($F(3,15)=4.45$, $p=0.02$) as well as a significant main effect for force ($F(3,15)=18.40$, $p<0.001$). Similarly, the ANOVA comparing HHFM-on and HHFM-off showed greater magnitudes for the HHFM-on condition ($F(1,5)=37.31$, $p=0.002$), a significant interaction ($F(3,15)=4.54$, $p=0.02$) and a significant main effect for force ($F(3,15)=15.11$, $p<0.001$).

4 Discussion

Our psychophysical experiments clearly show that percepts of force at both threshold and supra-threshold levels are rescaled when using the HHFM, demonstrating that the force magnification induced by the device is well perceived by human users. The perceptual force magnifications observed in the two experiments are less than the actual magnification, particularly in the force-estimation experiment. This loss of force magnification through perceptual transmission might be due to the friction observed in the custom solenoid. Two additional issues should also be noted in interpreting this result. First, the perceptual magnification was estimated here by a linear regression analysis, whereas the curves in Fig 6a were best fitted by power functions with exponents of 0.71 and 0.96, respectively, for the HHFM-on and HHFM-off data. Without considering such compressive nonlinearity in force perception, the magnification derived from the linear fitting of HHFM-on vs. HHFM-off data would be underestimated. Second, since the HHFM is pinch-held by the user as illustrated in Figs. 2 and 3, force perception is significantly influenced by the surface texture at the contact locations [12]. Essentially, the smoother the surface texture, the greater the grip force required and the more difficult it is to perceive the axial force. In the current prototype, the handle of the HHFM is the body of a syringe that has fine surface texture. This may contribute to the reduced perception of axial forces transmitted along the HHFM handle. In future research we will examine these issues further and revise the HHFM design accordingly to maximize the operator's perceptual magnification.

The following anecdotal observation surprised us. When pushing against the spring (see Fig. 2), we had expected the optimal motion to be that of just the fingertips moving the tool relative to the solenoid. Instead, we found that the most convincing sensation of magnified stiffness in the spring is achieved by moving the entire device, including the solenoid, with the muscles of the upper arm and shoulder. This makes little sense from a Newtonian point of view, since the device is only capable of generating forces between the solenoid and the fingertips. It indicates that force perception at the fingertips is influenced by sensorimotor integration between the fingers, hands, arms, and shoulders.

It is too early to predict exactly which clinical applications may prove most suitable for the HHFM, or to know what types of tool-tips will be most useful. At present, we are primarily considering applications in ophthalmological surgery. This is, in part, due to the authors' ongoing collaboration with ophthalmological surgeons in developing techniques for image guidance for eye surgery, but also because eye surgery is so clearly a realm in which many very delicate operations are performed. Two primary categories of eye surgery are procedures on the cornea and those on the retina. Corneal procedures are generally less delicate than retinal procedures, and are closer to the surface and therefore more accessible, but both corneal and retinal procedures are performed under the surgical microscope, involve extremely fine motor skills, and are often devoid of a useful sense of touch.

Corneal Surgery: Several corneal procedures are used to treat glaucoma, including *trabeculotomy* and *canaloplasty*, which create communication between the anterior chamber and Schlemm's canal, decreasing resistance to outflow. Trabeculotomy involves using a tiny blunt device to tear through the inner wall of Schlemm's canal and surrounding trabecular meshwork. Canaloplasty involves injecting viscoelastic material through a microcatheter along the entire 360° path of the canal and placing a stent suture. A third, experimental technique involves insertion of permanent stents into the canal *ab interno*, bypassing the trabecular meshwork to permit aqueous humor direct access to Schlemm's canal. These manipulations could be aided by an enhanced sense of touch provided by HHFM-based tools. Another candidate is *keratectomy* to repair corneal dystrophies, scars, or damage from foreign bodies, as well as *Deep Anterior Lamellar Keratectomy* to treat the gradual bulging of the cornea into a conical shape. In this latter procedure, perforation of Descemet's membrane often leads to mandatory conversion to *Penetrating Keratoplasty* a more radical procedure. It may be that greater sensitivity to forces could prevent this. Finally, corneal transplant commonly involves a *Descemet's Stripping Automated Endothelial Keratoplasty* (DSAEK), which maintains the patient's own outer cornea, replacing just the inner portion with donor tissue inserted through a small slit. The procedure is extremely delicate, both in the actual transplantation and in the prior harvesting of the graft from the donor.

Retinal Surgery: Procedures on the retina are generally even more delicate than those in the cornea, and have the added constraint that the tool must first be inserted through the sclera to reach the retina. The particular procedures we are considering involve peeling one of several types of membranes off the retina. An *epiretinal membrane* (ERM) is a glial cell proliferation that can cause blurred or distorted central vision. After removing the vitreous, the surgeon scores the ERM with a barb and then pulls it up with forceps or a diamond-dusted scraper. Another type of membrane, the *internal limiting membrane* (ILM), is a naturally occurring extracellular matrix that guides axons during the formation of the retina but is not needed thereafter. It has been shown that removing the (ILM) increases the closure rate of holes in the macula (the highest resolution portion of the fovea) that can significantly impede vision. Observing a retinal surgeon remove such membranes from the retina with nothing but visual feedback is instructive as to what is possible freehand. In particular, extremely fine control of tiny motion is possible when stabilized by insertion of the hand-held tool through the sclera. Also critical is the position of the surgeon's hand resting on the patient. Clearly, forces generated within the hand are central to such fine motor control. In particular, the act of gently peeling a membrane away from the retina, preferably in one piece without tearing it, seems to be a good candidate for increased sensitivity to minute forces.

In the face of such extremely delicate procedures, the Model-1 prototype leaves much room for improvement. As mentioned above, magnifications only up to 5.8 are presently possible without instability. Higher magnification may be useful in microsurgery, and would likely be possible with the inclusion of differential and/or integral gain, using a classical Proportional-Integral-Differential (PID) controller. The present amplifier can send current either way through the solenoid, so that by using a bidirectional force sensor we will be able to test tools that pull, such as hooks, as well as push. It is theoretically possible to also magnify non-axial forces and even torques with the HHFM. The present location of the brace may make it difficult to efficiently produce such lateral forces at the tool tip. A certain amount of natural lateral force magnification is, in fact, already present at the fingertips, due to the relative lengths of the lever arms. However, it is clear that the alternate approach of using an external robotic arm (as described in the Introduction) would make such lateral forces and torques easier to generate. Other improvements to the HHFM, such as the production of multiple simultaneous forces, as between the tips of a forceps, are also candidates for inclusion in future prototypes.

It is likely that when extremely small forces are involved, the external robotic arm may be advantageous due to the added stability of a grounded platform. Conversely, patient movement relative to such a stationary platform may prove a serious problem, favoring smaller, truly telerobotic systems that brace against the patient to generate forces for micromanipulation, such as the HeartLander system for minimally invasive cardiac surgery [13]. In the spectrum of such devices, it may be that the HHFM is best suited for an intermediate range of forces, perhaps in the cornea or elsewhere in the body, where structures of the appropriate range of delicacy are targets for surgical procedures.

5 Conclusion

The major contribution of our work, we believe, is to provide a magnified sense of touch without requiring an external robotic arm. The force that was generated between the operator's hand and the floor by the robotic arm is replaced by a force generated between two locations on the operator's hand, freeing the design to permit a small, light, hand-held device. Such a device may be easier to manipulate and more practical to deploy in certain clinical settings, where fewer degrees of freedom and intermediate force sensitivity are acceptable trade-offs for greater flexibility and independence of operation.

Acknowledgments. This work was funded by a NIH K99 grant 5K99EB008710 and a William Kepler Whiteford Professorship at the University of Pittsburgh.

References

1. Galeotti, J., Sajjad, A., Wang, B., Kagemann, L., Shukla, G., Siegel, M., Wu, B., Klatzky, R., Wollstein, G., Schuman, J., Stetten, G.: The OCT penlight: In-situ image guidance for microsurgery, SPIE Medical Imaging, paper #7625-1 (2010)
2. Bethea, B., Okamura, A., Kitagawa, M., Fitton, T., Cattaneo, S., Gott, V., Baumgartner, W., Yuy, D.: Application of Haptic Feedback to Robotic Surgery. J. Laparoendosc Adv. Surg. Tech. A 14(3), 191–195 (2004)
3. Kuchenbecker, K.J., Gewirtz, J., McMahan, W., Standish, D., Martin, P., Bohren, J., Mendoza, P.J., Lee, D.I.: VerroTouch: High-frequency acceleration feedback for telerobotic surgery. In: Kappers, A.M.L., van Erp, J.B.F., Bergmann Tiest, W.M., van der Helm, F.C.T. (eds.) EuroHaptics 2010. LNCS, vol. 6191, pp. 189–196. Springer, Heidelberg (2010)
4. Salcudean, S.E., Yan, J.: Motion scaling teleoperating system with force feedback suitable for microsurgery, U.S. Patent 5,382,885 (1995)
5. Salcudean, S.E., Yan, J.: Towards a Force-Reflecting Motion-Scaling System for Microsurgery. In: IEEE International Conference on Robotics and Automation, San Diego, California (1994)
6. Taylor, R., Barnes, A., Kumar, R., Gupta, P., Wang, Z., Jensen, P., Whitcomb, L.: A steady-hand robotic system for microsurgical augmentation. In: Taylor, C., Colchester, A. (eds.) MICCAI 1999. LNCS, vol. 1679, pp. 1031–1041. Springer, Heidelberg (1999)
7. Fleming, I., Balicki, M., Koo, J., Iordachita, I.I., Mitchell, B., Handa, J., Hager, G.D., Taylor, R.: Cooperative robot assistant for retinal microsurgery. In: Metaxas, D., Axel, L., Fichtinger, G., Székely, G. (eds.) MICCAI 2008, Part II. LNCS, vol. 5242, pp. 543–550. Springer, Heidelberg (2008)
8. Tabars, J., MacLachlan, R., Ettensohn, C., Riviere, C.: Cell Micromanipulation with an Active Handheld Micromanipulator. In: 32nd Annual International Conference of the IEEE EMBS, Buenos Aires, Argentina (2010)
9. Solazzi, M., Frisoli, A., Bergamasco, M.: Design of a Novel Finger Haptic Interface for Contact and Orientation Display. In: IEEE Haptics Symposium, Waltham, Massachusetts (March 25-26, 2010)
10. Hollis, R.L., Salcudean, E.: Lorentz Levitation Technology: A New Approach to Fine Motion Robotics, Teleoperation, Haptic Interfaces, and Vibration Isolation. In: 5th International Symposium on Robotics Research, Hidden Valley, PA, October 1-4 (1993)
11. Stevens, S.S.: Psychophysics: Introduction to its Perceptual, Neural, and Social Prospects. John Wiley, New York (1975)
12. Flanagan, J.R., Wing, A.M.: Effects of surface texture and grip force on the discrimination of hand-held loads. Perception & Psychophysics 59, 111–118 (1997)
13. Ota, T., Patronik, N., Riviere, C., Zenati, M.A.: Percutaneous Subxiphoid Access to the Epicardium Using a Miniature Crawling Robotic Device. Innovations 1(5), 227–231 (2006)

PS-GANS: A Patient-Specific, Gravity Assisted Navigation System for Acetabular Cup Placement

Guoyan Zheng[1], Santiago Echeverri[2], Weiguo Xie[1], and Lutz-Peter Nolte[1]

[1] Institute for Surgical Technology and Biomechanics, University of Bern, CH-3014, Bern, Switzerland
guoyan.zheng@ieee.org
[2] Swisss Ortho Clinic, Lausanne, Switzerland

Abstract. In this paper we propose a new system that allows reliable acetabular cup placement when the THA is operated in lateral approach. Conceptually it combines the accuracy of computer-generated patient-specific morphology information with an easy-to-use mechanical guide, which effectively uses natural gravity as the angular reference. The former is achieved by using a statistical shape model-based 2D-3D reconstruction technique that can generate a scaled, patient-specific 3D shape model of the pelvis from a single conventional anteroposterior (AP) pelvic X-ray radiograph. The reconstructed 3D shape model facilitates a reliable and accurate co-registration of the mechanical guide with the patient's anatomy in the operating theater. We validated the accuracy of our system by conducting experiments on placing seven cups to four pelvises with different morphologies. Taking the measurements from an image-free navigation system as the ground truth, our system showed an average accuracy of 2.1 ± 0.7^o for inclination and an average accuracy of 1.2 ± 1.4^o for anteversion.

1 Introduction

Total hip arthroplasty (THA) is one of the most frequent orthopaedic surgical interventions. Proper positioning, in particular angulation of the acetabular cup, is the essential of improving the success of total hip arthroplasty. Previous studies [1][2][3][4][5][6] demonstrate that higher rates of pelvis osteolysis and component migration have all been well associated with the malpositioning of the acetabular component, and surgical experience indicates that improper orientation of the acetabular component in terms of anteversion and inclination is the major cause of dislocation. As the risk of dislocation is significantly higher in those who have already experienced dislocation or after revision surgery [6], obtaining proper cup orientation during primary surgery is crucial.

Optimal ranges for angular cup position in terms of anteversion and inclination of the acetabular component have been extensively debated in the literature. Several so-called safe zones have been suggested. Lewinnek et al. described a safe zone of 5° to 25° for anteversion and 30° to 50° for inclination [5]. They found

R.H. Taylor and G.-Z. Yang (Eds.): IPCAI 2011, LNCS 6689, pp. 101–112, 2011.

that acetabular cups placed outside this safe zone were approximately four times as likely to dislocate. Consequently optimal cup positioning requires that the surgeon attains adequate and reproducible angulations of the acetabular component with respect to the patient's individual pelvic morphology.

State of the art mechanical guides, which are used in the vast majority of THAs are easy to handle but cannot be registered to the individual pelvic morphology. Angular orientation is gained from reference objects in space fixed coordinates and may be corrected/optimized through the surgeon's expert knowledge. A study conducted by DiGioia et al. [7], in which they used navigation technology to evaluate the performance of mechanical guides, found that 78% of the inserted cups would have been implanted outside the safe zone as suggested by Lewinnek et al [5].

The search for alternatives was unsuccessful until modern optoelectronic-tracking/robotic technology was introduced to the field of orthopaedics. Previously, a variety of image-based and image-free so-called navigation systems have been introduced for THA [8][9][10][11][12][13], which for the first time allowed co-registration of the patient's pelvic morphology. Despite encouraging results of smaller clinical trials and an early widespread enthusiasm, some drawbacks of navigation technology have been identified, which prevent their wide spread use in clinical routine. Current criticism focuses on: (a) significant investments required for acquisition and running costs for maintenance, and use (training of users, additional operating room (OR) time, disposable markers, etc.); (b) all navigation systems proposed to date, no matter what image modality is used, have difficulty when the THA is operated in lateral approach, which is the approach of choice for more than 80% of THAs worldwide [13]; (c) the steep learning curve and the system complexities, which may result in $10-20\%$ failure cases [12]; (d) optoelectronic tracking technology used in most navigation systems requires a straight line-of-sight, which is often difficult to maintain during surgery without paying additional efforts and time; (e) CT-based systems require CT scan, usually not performed for diagnosis, generating unnecessary radiation exposure to the patient and significant additional cost; (f) for image-free navigation systems, significant intra- and inter-observer variability caused by variations during digitization of the anatomical landmarks, especially the one in the pubic region, were observed [14]; and (g) fluoroscopy-based navigation systems [12] have the advantage of eliminating a CT scan and achieving an equivalent accuracy. However, such a technology requires calibration of the image intensifier and it was judged to be too cumbersome and time-consuming to intra-operatively manipulate the C-arm device for multiple image acquisition [12].

Recently, several groups [15][16][17] described methods to use the constant direction of the force of gravity as a reference in THA. Asayama et al.[15][16] introduced a three-direction indicator to control intra-operative pelvic motion during THAs. The three-direction indicator incorporates a digital compass with two goniometers, as well as a pendulum and target apparatus. It allows for controlling only pelvic motion by measuring the three-dimensional (3D) angle formed by the gravitational direction and the Steinmann pin inserted into the iliac bone to fix the direction indicator. No control of acetabular cup placement was considered with this device. Echeverri et al. [17] described a gravity assisted system to control both the pelvic motion and the acetabular component placement. Like any other mechanical guide, this system is simple to use, but it is also highly flawed. This is due to the fact that the alignment system developed by Echeverri et al. was placed in a fixed orientation relative to the shaft of a cup placement instrument, which in the best case scenario can be understood as being calibrated with respect to the morphology of a fixed pelvis without considering the morphological difference between the future pelvis to be navigated and the fixed pelvis used for calibration. It simply does not work due to the inherent morphological variations in human being. A recent simulation study of this device on 48 patient data revealed a maximum anteversion error of as high as 15° [18].

To address the limitations in the existing gravity-based systems, we developed a new gravity assisted navigation system termed as "Patient-specific, Gravity Assisted Navigation System" or "PS-GANS" in abbreviation. Conceptually it combines the accuracy of computer-generated patient-specific morphology information with an easy-to-use mechanical guide, which effectively uses natural gravity as the angular reference. Unlike the existing gravity-based systems, our system allows for calibration of the mechanical guide with respect to the patient-specific morphology, which is obtained by using a statistical shape model-based 2D-3D reconstruction technique that can generate a scaled, patient-specific 3D shape model of the pelvis from a single conventional anteroposterior (AP) X-ray radiograph. The reconstructed 3D shape model facilitates a reliable and accurate co-registration of the mechanical guide with the patient's anatomy in the operating theatre.

2 Materials and Methods

2.1 Notations

Throughout the paper, we always establish a local coordinate system of a rigid body on a local reference plane of the entity. Thus, without explicitly stating, we always name the local coordinate system after the local reference plane. Furthermore, a vector $\mathtt{v}$ that is defined in a local coordinate system X will be noted as $\mathtt{v}^{\mathtt{X}}$. But if we would like to know the axis $\mathtt{v}$ of a local coordinate system $\mathtt{X}$ in another local coordinate system $\mathtt{Y}$, we will note it as $\mathtt{v}_{\mathtt{X}}^{\mathtt{Y}}$. A rigid body transformation from a local coordinate system $\mathtt{X}$ to another local coordinate system $\mathtt{Y}$ will be noted as $\mathtt{T}_{\mathtt{X}}^{\mathtt{Y}}$. The inverse of this transformation will be recorded as $\mathtt{T}_{\mathtt{Y}}^{\mathtt{X}}$. As in most of the time, we are only interested in knowing the orientation of a vector in a local coordinate system, knowing rotational part $\mathtt{R}_{\mathtt{X}}^{\mathtt{Y}}$ of the rigid body transformation $\mathtt{T}_{\mathtt{X}}^{\mathtt{Y}}$ is enough for our purpose.

2.2 System Overview

Our system requires three Bull's-eye bubble levels, as shown in Fig. 1. The first one is called witness bubble level that is fixed on the iliac crest and is designed

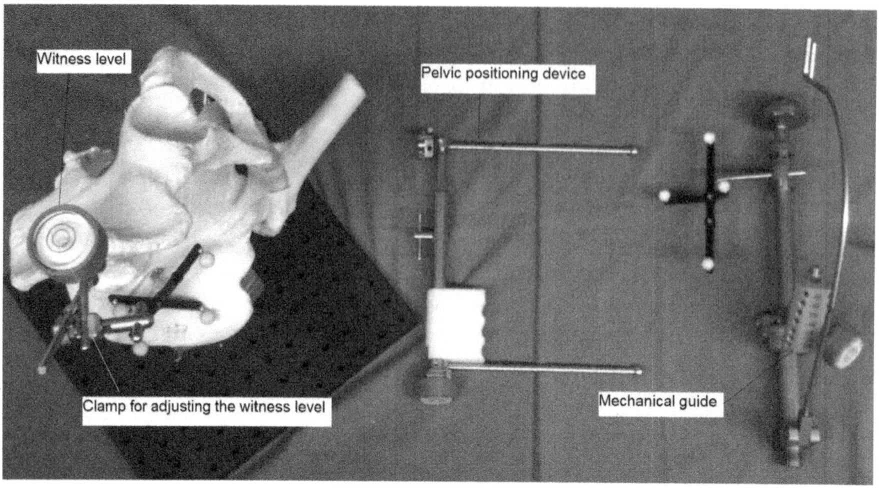

Fig. 1. An overview of the PS-GANS system

together with the one on the pelvic positioning device to place the pelvis to strict lateral decubitus. As soon as the pelvis is placed at strict lateral decubitus by using the pelvic positioning device, one can adjust a standard clamp to set the witness level's bubble to the center and move away the pelvic positioning device (see below for details). The witness level then acts as a witness, identifying the strict lateral decubitus position of the pelvis throughout the operation. The third one is called the instrument bubble level that is placed on a mechanical guide that is rigidly attached to the cup placement instrument for controlling cup orientation to the desired anteversion and inclination. Please keep it in mind that all the passive markers appeared in Fig. 1 is only for our validation purpose and are not required to use our system.

2.3 Coordinate Systems

Before we describe the details about how the patient-specific system calibration is done, we would like to first present a summary of all four local reference planes as well as their associated local coordinate systems that will be used in the calibration. See Fig. 2(a) for an overview.

Jamaraz et al. [10] introduced the Anterior Pelvic Plane (APP) concept for measuring anteversion and inclination of the acetabular cup in their computer assisted acetabular cup placement system. The APP is a reference plane of the human pelvis and thus, allowing the exact definition of a corresponding 3D local coordinate system as shown in Fig. 2(a). It is based on three landmarks: bilateral Anterior Superior Iliac Spines (ASIS) and the geometric center of two pubic tubercles. The APP x-axis points to the patient's operating side, parallel with the line between the iliac spine points. The y-axis points inferior. The angular

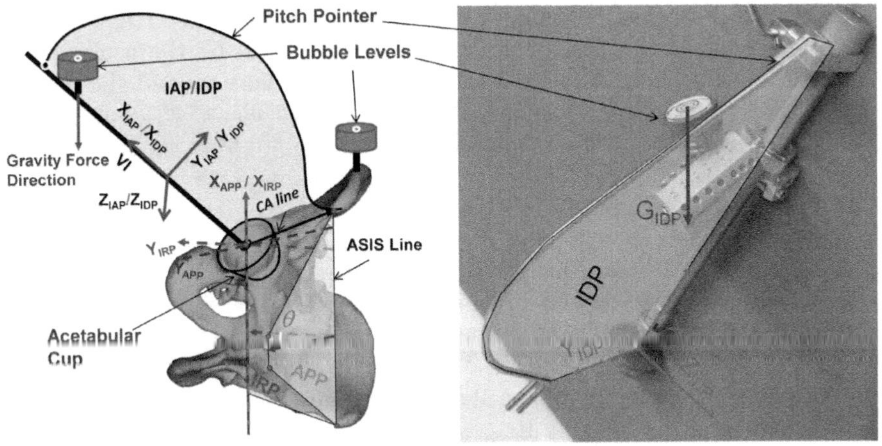

(a) (b)

Fig. 2. (a) Schematic view of the relationship between the APP, the IRP, and the IAP (IDP) when the cup is placed in the desired orientation; (b) The mechanical guide attached to the cup placement instrument and the definition of the IDP

orientation of the acetabular component can be directly put into relation to the APP.

It is difficult, if it is not impossible, to locate the orientation of the APP without using a positional tracking device, largely due to the difficulty in mechanically aligning the geometric center of two pubic tubercles. In this work, we propose and use a new reference plane that is called Intra-operative Reference Plane (IRP), which is defined by two lines that can be mechanically aligned with the design of our system: the line connecting the bilateral ASISs (we named it as the ASIS line) and the line CA from the cup center of the operating side to the ASIS of the operating side (we named it as the CA line). Similar to how we establish a 3D local coordinate system on the APP, we also establish a 3D local coordinate system on the IRP, as shown in Fig. 2(a), where we translate the origins of both coordinate systems to the acetabular center of the operating side. As we are only interested in the orientation of the acetabular component, such a translation does not affect our analysis and computation below. The x-axis of the IRP local coordinate system has the same orientation as the x-axis of the APP local coordinate system, while the y-axis of the IRP local coordinate system is chose to be a vector that is inside the IRP and perpendicular to the x-axis. The z-axis of the IRP local coordinate system can be computed from the cross product of the x-axis and the y-axis of the IRP local coordinate system.

The so-called Instrument Design Plane (IDP) is a plane that is defined by the design of the mechanical guide as shown in Fig. 2(b). Physically, it is defined by the instrument axis and a curved metal rod called the pitch pointer, as shown in Fig. 2(b). The pitch pointer is calibrated to be always inside the IDP and to be freely rotated around a fixed axis at the distal end of the cup placement instrument. We could establish a local coordinate system on the IDP as follows. The origin of this local coordinate system is chosen to be the center of the attached cup; the x-axis is chosen to be the instrument axis and the y-axis is defined as a vector that is inside the IDP and perpendicular to the x-axis. The z-axis of the IDP local coordinate system can be computed from the cross product of the x-axis and the y-axis of the IDP local coordinate system.

Given a desired orientation of the cup (e.g., a typical desired orientation of the cup is 20° anteversion and 45° inclination with respect to the APP), we can construct a virtual instrument axis with respect to the APP of the pelvis using the method introduced by Murray [19] and we call its direction as VI^{APP}. This axis together with the CA line define the Instrument Alignment Plane (IAP), to which the IDP should be aligned in order to place the cup in the desired orientation using the method described below. Thus, similar to how we define a local coordinate system on the IDP, we also establish a local coordinate system on the IAP (see Fig. 2(a) for a schematic view of how the local coordinate system of the IAP is established). More specifically, we take the virtual instrument axis as the x-axis of the IAP local coordinate system. The y-axis is defined as a vector that is inside the IAP and perpendicular to the x-axis.

2.4 System Calibration

System calibration here means to define the orientation of the instrument bubble level as shown in Fig. 2(b) with respect to the local coordinate system of the IDP for a given pelvis whose morphology is known (the exact morphological information that our system requires will be described below), so that when all system requirements are satisfied (see below for the details about our system requirements) and when the bubble of the instrument level is oriented to the center, the axis of the cup placement instrument should be aligned with the virtual instrument axis that is constructed according to the desired orientation of the cup.

Without loss of generality, let's assume that the x-axis of the IRP of the given pelvis is $[1\,0\,0]^T$, the y-axis of the IRP is $[0\,1\,0]^T$, and the z-axis is $[0\,0\,1]^T$. As the morphology of this pelvis is given, we assume that we know the angle θ between its APP and its IRP, and we further assume that we know the orientation of the CA line in the local coordinate system of the IRP, which is defined as CA^{IRP}. Using angle θ, we can find the rotation between the local coordinate system of the IRP and the local coordinate system of the APP, R^{IRP}_{APP}, and the inverse rotation R^{APP}_{IRP} as well. With rotation matrix R^{IRP}_{APP}, one can transform the vector VI^{APP} from the local coordinate system of APP to the local coordinate system of IRP and denote it as VI^{IRP}.

$$VI^{IRP} = R^{IRP}_{APP}(\theta) \cdot VI^{APP} \tag{1}$$

When our system would be used for the navigation of the cup placement, additionally we require that: A) the pelvis should be placed in strict lateral decubitus, which means that the ASIS line should be parallel to the constant direction of the force of gravity (but with opposite direction). This is realized intra-operatively

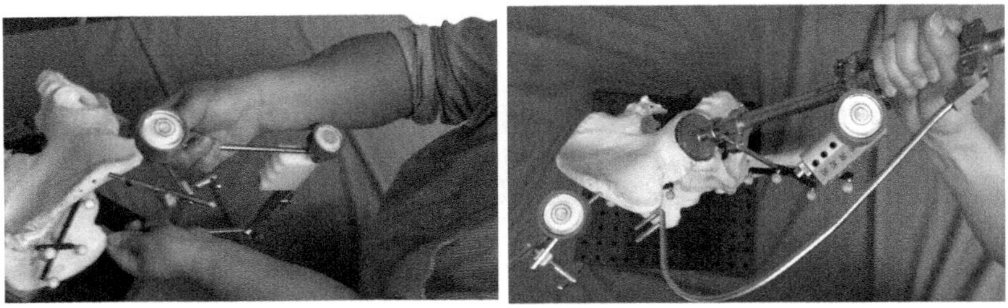

(a) (b)

Fig. 3. (a) This image shows how to use the pelvic positioning device to place the pelvis in strict lateral decubitus and then to set the witness level at zero; (b) this image illustrates the touch of the pitch pointer on the ASIS of the operating side during cup placement navigation

by using the pelvic positioning device and the witness level, as shown in Fig. 3(a), following the procedure introduced by Echeverri et al. [17]; and B) the pitch pointer should touch on the ASIS of the operating side of the pelvis, as shown in Fig. 3(b). As only a thin layer of soft tissue exists on top of the ASIS of the operating side, this landmark can be easily palpatable by a surgeon [13].

According to the requirement A), the constant direction G of the force of gravity in the IRP coordinate system can now be represented as:

$$G^{IRP} = [-1\ 0\ 0]^T \tag{2}$$

When the cup would be placed in the desired orientation by the cup placement instrument and at the same time when the requirement B) is satisfied, the IDP would be aligned with the IAP (see Fig. 2(a) for details). Thus, at this moment, the orientations of the axes of the local coordinate system of the IDP (or the IAP, as the IDP is aligned with the IAP) with respect to the local coordinate system of the IRP of the pelvis are,

$$\begin{cases} x_{IDP}^{IRP} = VI^{IRP} \\ z_{IDP}^{IRP} = \frac{VI^{IRP} \times CA^{IRP}}{|VI^{IRP} \times CA^{IRP}|} \\ y_{IDP}^{IRP} = z_{IDP}^{IRP} \times x_{IDP}^{IRP} \end{cases} \tag{3}$$

where "×" means the cross product of two vectors.

And the rotation from the local coordinate system of the IRP to the local coordinate system of the IDP is:

$$R_{IRP}^{IDP} = [R_{IDP}^{IRP}]^T = [x_{IDP}^{IRP}\ y_{IDP}^{IRP}\ z_{IDP}^{IRP}]^T \tag{4}$$

We thus can transform the constant direction of the force of gravity from the local coordinate system of the IRP to the local coordinate system of the IDP,

$$G^{IDP} = R_{IRP}^{IDP} \cdot G^{IRP} \tag{5}$$

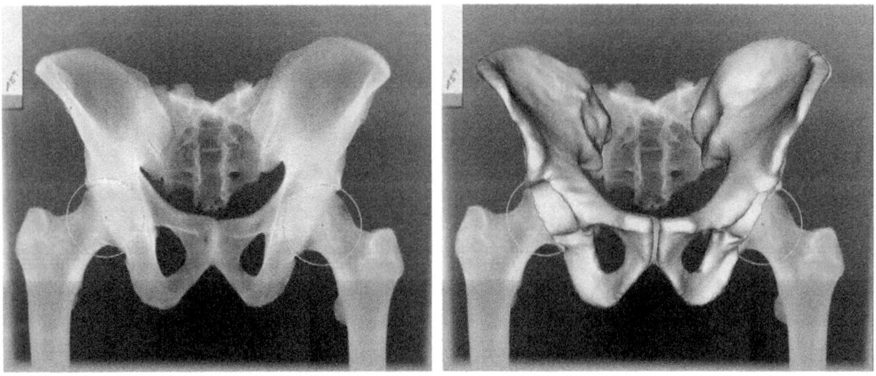

Fig. 4. One convention AP pelvic X-ray radiograph of a pelvis used in our experiment (left) and the model reconstructed from the radiograph (right)

We could then further compute the three angles between G^{IDP} with all three axes of the local coordinate system of the IDP. Given an arbitrary fixation point on the cup placement instrument, these three angles will uniquely determine an alignment direction along which the instrument bubble level should be placed such that when the bubble is placed to the center by orienting the cup placement instrument and its attached level and when the above two requirements are satisfied, the cup will be placed in the desired orientation. This principle has been used to design a mechanical guide as shown in Fig. 2(b) and Fig. 3(b). The mechanical guide has an intra-operatively exchangeable steel block with a set of pre-manufactured holes, where each hole defines an alignment orientation along which the instrument bubble level should be placed. Intra-operatively, according to the desired cup orientation and the patient-specific morphological information, the surgeon can choose the right steel block with the correctly oriented hole to place the instrument bubble level.

2.5 2D-3D X-Ray Radiograph Reconstruction-Based Morphological Information Derivation

As clearly indicated in the above calibration procedure, the system calibration is a patient-specific task. Given a desired cup orientation, the exact decomposition of the constant direction of the force of gravity with respect to the three axes of the local coordinate system of the IDP depends on two patient-specific morphological parameters: a) the angle θ between the APP and the IRP of the pelvis; and b) the orientation of the CA line in the local coordinate system of the IRP of the pelvis. Both parameters can be easily obtained from a CT or a MRI scan. However, these have the disadvantages that they are expensive, time-consuming and/or induce high-radiation doses to the patient. More importantly, they are not part of the standard treatment loop of every patient in clinical routine. In

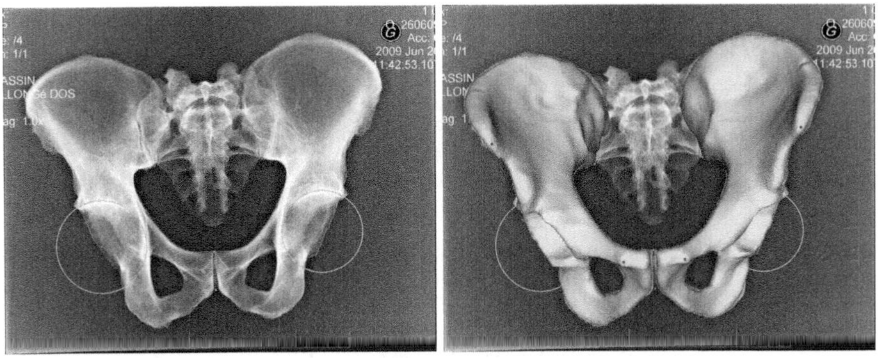

Fig. 5. Another example of the single image based 2D-3D reconstruction of a pelvis used in our experiment which has different morphology from the one shown in Fig. 4. Left: a convention AP pelvic X-ray radiograph of the pelvis; right: the model reconstructed from the radiograph.

this paper, we propose to use a statistically deformable 2D-3D reconstruction technique [20], which can reconstruct a scaled, patient-specific 3D model from a single conventional AP pelvic X-ray radiograph based on a statistical shape model of the pelvis. The reconstructed model can then be used to extract all the required morphological parameters. Fig. 4 shows one example of applying this technique to reconstruct a 3D surface model of the pelvis from a conventional AP pelvic X-ray radiograph. Another example of the single image based 2D-3D reconstruction of a pelvis used in our experiment which has different morphology from the one shown in Fig. 4 is presented in Fig. 5. As we are only interested in the angular or orientational information, a scaled, patient-specific 3D model will be accurate enough for our purpose.

3 Experiments and Results

We designed and conducted two studies on placing seven cups to four pelvises with different morphologies (four left sides and three right sides) to validate the accuracy of the present system. As all the pelvises were dry bones, we implemented an image-free navigation system following the principles introduced by Dorr et al. [13] to get the ground truth measurement for each experiment. Every time when the bubble of the instrument level is placed at the center, we recorded the measurements of the image-free navigation system. For all the experiments, the desired cup orientation is set to be 45° inclination and 20° anteversion.

For the first study, we acquired one conventional AP X-ray radiograph for each pelvis. The morphological information extracted from a surface model that was reconstructed from the X-ray radiograph of the associated pelvis was used to calibrate our system. This study was designed to validate the accuracy of the present system in placing the acetabular cups to different pelvises with different

Table 1. Difference between the desired cup orientation and the cup orientation actually achieved by the present system

angle	B_01, L	B_01, R	B_02, L	B_02, R	B_03, L	B_03, R	B_04, L	Mean
anteversion (^{o})	0.1	0.4	0.8	3.4	0.2	3.0	0.6	1.2 ± 1.4
inclination (^{o})	1.6	1.8	1.8	2.2	1.4	3.4	2.6	2.1 ± 0.7

Table 2. Difference between the desired cup orientation and the actually achieved one when different X-ray radiographs were used

angle	Img_01	Img_02	Img_03	Img_04	Img_05	Mean
anteversion (^{o})	1.4	0.8	0.7	1.1	0.0	0.8 ± 0.5
inclination (^{o})	2.3	1.9	2.3	2.0	2.2	2.1 ± 0.2

morphologies. For this purpose, every time when the bubble of the instrument level was placed at the center and when both system requirements were satisfied, the recorded measurements from the image-free navigation system were compared to the desired cup orientation. Table-1 summarizes the placement errors where an average accuracy of 2.1 ± 0.7^o was found for inclination and an average accuracy of 1.2 ± 1.4^o was found for anteversion.

The second study was designed to validate how sensitive the present system is to the orientation of the pelvis with respect to the X-ray table during image acquisition. For this purpose, one pelvis (B_04) was chosen and the pelvis was placed in different orientations with respect to the X-ray plate. Starting from an initial position, which we defined as the 0° position, we tilted the pelvis around the acetabular center line in one direction with an incremental interval of 5° until 20° and at each orientation we acquired one X-ray radiograph. We thus obtained five X-ray radiographs of the same pelvis. We then reconstructed a surface model of the pelvis from each X-ray radiograph and used the reconstructed model to derive morphological parameters for the instrument calibration. Based on the calibration, we performed the similar experiments as we did in the first study. Table-2 shows the placement errors when different X-ray radiographs were used to derive the patient-specific morphological parameters.

4 Discussions and Conclusions

In this paper, we presented a patient-specific, gravity assisted navigation system for high-precision placement of acetabular cup for THA operated in lateral approach. It starts with a 2D-3D reconstruction of a scaled, patient-specific 3D surface model of the pelvis from one conventional AP pelvis X-ray radiograph. The reconstructed 3D model facilitates a reliable and accurate co-registration of a gravity assisted mechanical guide with the patient's anatomy in the operating theater. We validated the accuracy of our system by conducting experiments on placing seven cups to four pelvises with different morphologies. The experimental results demonstrated the efficacy of the present system.

The rationale of using the measurements of an image-free navigation system as the ground truth in our experiment should be discussed. Previously, several studies [21][22][23] have suggested that CT-based solutions seem to be the most reliable method for non-invasive post-operative assessment of the acetabular cup orientation with experienced and trained observers. Probably this is true for those studies where there are no direct bone access to the anatomical landmarks that are required to precisely calculate the post-operative cup orientation. In such a situation, all the required landmarks have to be digitized percutaneously, which lead to errors in determining the cup orientation. In contrast, in the present study, all pelvises used in our experiment are dry bones. We can thus do direct bone digitization with our image-free navigation system, which may result in more accurate ground truth than the CT-based method according to what have been reported by Lin et al. [24].

Our system offers several advantages in comparison to other existing systems. First, instead of using a positional tracker, whose price ranges from several thousand Euros to dozens of thousand Euros, our system uses a mechanical guide with Bull's eye-bubble level indicators, taking advantage of the constant direction of the natural gravity force as a globally available reference for acetabular cup placement. Second, unlike most previously introduced mechanical alignment units, our system allows for a calibration with respect to the patient's individualized morphology. Furthermore, in our system the patient-specific morphological information is derived from a 3D surface model of the pelvis that is reconstructed from a conventional AP X-ray radiograph using a statistically deformable 2D-3D registration approach. No CT/MRI scan is required. Our system is completely integrated with the standard treatment protocol.

References

1. Kahn, A.M.A., Brakenbury, P.H., et al.: Dislocation following total hip replacement. J. Bone Joint Surg. 63B, 214–218 (1981)
2. McCollum, D.E., Gray, W.J.G.: Dislocation after Total Hip Arthroplasty. Causes and Prevention. Clin. Orthop. 261, 159–170 (1990)
3. Sarmiento, A., Ebramzadeh, E., et al.: Cup containment and orientation in cemented total hip arthoplasties. J. Bone Joint Surg. 72B, 960–996 (1990)
4. Bader, R.J., Steinhauser, E., Willmann, G., Gradinger, R.: The effects of implant position, design and wear on the range of motion after total hip arthroplasty. Hip International 11, 80–90 (2001)
5. Lewinnek, G.E., Lewis, J.L., et al.: Dislocation after total hip-replacement arthroplasties. J. Bone Joing Surg. 60A, 217–220 (1978)
6. Kotwal, R.S., Ganapathi, M., John, A., Maheson, M., Jones, S.A.: Outcome of treatment for dislocation after primary total hip replacement. J. Bone Joint Surg. 91B, 321–326 (2009)
7. Digioia III, A.M., Jaramaz, B., Plakseychuk, A.Y., et al.: Comparison of a mechanical acetabular alignment guide with computer placement of the socket. J. Arthroplasty 17, 359–364 (2002)

8. DiGioia III, A.M., et al.: The Otto Aufranc Award: image-guided navigation system to measure intraoperatively acetabular implant alignment. Clin. Orthop. 355, 8–22 (1998)
9. Bargar, W.L., et al.: Primary and revision total hip replacement using the Robodoc systems. Clin. Orthop. 354, 82–91 (1998)
10. Jaramaz, B., et al.: Computer assisted measurement of cup placement in total hip replacement. Clin. Orthop. 354, 70–81 (1998)
11. Taylor, R.H., et al.: Computer-integrated revision total hip replacement surgery: concept and preliminary results. Med. Image Anal. 3, 301–319 (1999)
12. Zheng, G., et al.: A hybrid CT-free navigation system for total hip arthroplasty. Comput. Aided Surg. 7, 129–145 (2002)
13. Dorr, L.D., et al.: Development of imageless computer navigation for acetabular component position in total hip replacement. Iowa Orthop. J. 25, 1–9 (2005)
14. Spencer, J.M., et al.: Computer navigation of the acetabular component: a cadaver reliability study. J. Bone Joint Surg. 88B, 972–975 (2006)
15. Asayama, I., et al.: Intraoperative pelvic motion in total hip Arthroplasty. J. Arthroplasty 19, 992–997 (2004)
16. Ezoe, M., et al.: Pelvic motion during total hip Arthroplasty with translateral and posterolateral approaches. J. Orthop. Sci. 10, 167–172 (2005)
17. Echeverri, S., et al.: Reliable acetabular cup orientation with a new gravity-assisted guidance system. J. Arthroplasty 21, 413–419 (2006)
18. Dong, X., et al.: Acetabular cup orientation using a statistical data based calibration table. In: Proc. of CAOS 2008, Hongkong, China, June 4-7, pp. 262–265 (2008)
19. Murray, D.W.: The definition and measurement of acetabular orientation. J. Bone Joint Surg. 75, 228–232 (1993)
20. Zheng, G.: Statistically deformable 2D/3D registration for estimating post-operative cup orientation from a single standard X-ray radiograph. Annals of Biomedical Engineering 38, 2910–2927 (2010)
21. Arai, N., et al.: Minimal radioation dose computered tomography for measurement of cup orientation in total hip arthroplasty. Journal of Arthroplasty 25, 263–267 (2010)
22. Beckmann, J., et al.: Cup positioning in THA: current status and pitfalls. A systematic evaluation of the literature. Arch. Orthop. Trauma Surg. 129, 863–872 (2009)
23. Kalteis, T., et al.: Position of the acetabular cup - accuracy of radiographic calculation compared to CT-based measurement. Eur. J. Radiol. 58, 294–300 (2006)
24. Lin, F., et al.: Validation of a computer navigation system and a CT method for determination of the orientation of implanted acetabular cup in total hip arthroplasty: a cadaver study. Clinical Biomechanics 23, 1004–1011 (2008)

Correlating Clinical Scores with Anatomical Electrodes Locations for Assessing Deep Brain Stimulation

Florent Lalys[1,2,3], Claire Haegelen[1,2,3,4], Alexandre Abadie[1,2,3], and Pierre Jannin[1,2,3]

[1] INSERM, U746, Faculty of Medicine CS 34317, F-35043 Rennes, France
[2] INRIA, VisAGeS Unit/Project, F-35042 Rennes, France
[3] University of Rennes I, CNRS, UMR 6074, IRISA, F-35042 Rennes, France
[4] Department of Neurosurgery, Pontchaillou University Hospital, F-35043 Rennes, France

Abstract. Movement disorders in patients with Parkinson's disease may require functional surgery, when medical therapy isn't effective. In Deep Brain Stimulation (DBS), electrodes are implanted within the brain to stimulate deep structures such as SubThalamic Nucleus (STN). This paper describes successive steps for constructing digital atlases gathering patient's location of electrode contacts and clinical scores. Three motor and three neuro-psychological scores were integrated in the study. Correlations between active contacts localization and clinical data were carried out using an adapted Hierarchical Ascendant Classification and have enabled the extraction of clusters aiming to suggest optimum sites for therapeutic STN DBS. The postero-superior region has been found to be effective for motor score improvement whereas the antero-inferior region revealed noticeable neuro-psychological scores deterioration. Comparison with existing results has shown that such atlases are very promising for understanding phenomena better.

Keywords: Deep Brain Stimulation, digital atlases, subthalamic nucleus, Parkinson disease.

1 Introduction

Parkinson's disease (PD) is recognized as one of the most common neurological disorders, affecting 1% of people older than 60 years. The pathology is an age-related deterioration of certain nerve systems, which affects the patient's movement, balance, and muscle control. Major symptoms are indeed characterized by abnormalities of motor functions, several of which predominate, but all do not necessarily occur in all individuals. While these symptoms related to PD can be treated with medication therapy, few patients have side effects or treatments for which it is not effective. In such cases, Deep Brain Stimulation (DBS) [1] might be necessary, according to strict patient inclusion criteria. The target for DBS in Parkinson's disease has been moved from the ventro-lateral thalamic nucleus (Vlc) to the medial global pallidus (Gpm) and the Sub-Thalamic Nucleus (STN). Among these three deep brain structures, the STN became the mean target of high-frequency DBS in patients with PD and severe disabled symptoms [2]. Even if STN DBS has proved its efficiency for motor symptoms improvement, several studies have reported adverse-events after DBS surgery

R.H. Taylor and G.-Z. Yang (Eds.): IPCAI 2011, LNCS 6689, pp. 113–121, 2011.

affecting cognitive functions, emotion or behavior [3,4,5]. It remains interrogations about contacts location that provide the largest motor improvement while producing the least clinical side effects.

Preoperative definition of the target is based on the relief of symptoms and results of previous implantations only. Its precise localization from patient images is unfeasible mainly due to contrast and spatial resolutions limitations. Consequently, the surgeon needs additional information and knowledge for indirect identification of such small-targeted structures. Some are explicit such as anatomical atlases adapted to the patient images thanks to image registration. Some are implicit knowledge, such as the one acquired from learning, literature, and previous surgical cases. Different strategies have recently studied methods for making explicit this implicit information and knowledge. The concept of probabilistic functional atlases has been introduced [6]. After a step of normalisation within a common space, effective contacts are linked to a large panel of parameters acquired during the various stages of the procedure. The spatial normalisation allows performing retrospective studies, where statistical techniques are used to study anatomical or functional variability between patients. Response to stimulation, electro-physiological recordings, and clinical scores related to motor or cognitive evolution are all possible information that can be integrated in such atlases [7,8,9,10]. This fusion of information permits to understand functional organization within deep brain structures that helps for the identification of the optimal zone of therapy.

As far as we know, no functional atlases were proposed yet for representing the relationships between the anatomy and a large panel of clinical scores. While most of these atlases are using a single motor score for modelling the global outcome of the patient, we proposed in this paper to extend this research by adding motor and neuropsychological scores. We thus introduce the concept of anatomo-clinical atlases and describe the methods for their computation.

2 Materials and Methods

In this study, the objective was to correlate anatomical position of electrode contacts with clinical outcomes in STN DBS. After an automatic segmentation of electrode contacts for each patient, the crucial step was to perform an accurate patient-to-template registration, allowing expressing contacts coordinates in a common reference space. Then the integration of clinical scores obtained pre and post-operatively permitted the extraction of representative anatomo-clinical clusters. We describe in this section every stage of our procedure, from the extraction of electrode's contacts to the creation of atlases.

2.1 Data

The study population consisted of 23 patients (10 women and 13 men, mean age 60 years old) with idiopathic PD who had bilateral STN DBS according to selected inclusion criteria at the University Hospital of Rennes (France). Patients had preoperative 3-T T1-weighted MR (1 mm x 1 mm x 1 mm, Philips Medical Systems), pre and post-operative CT scans (0.44 mm x 0.44 mm x 0.6 mm in post-operative acquisitions and 0.5 mm x 0.5 mm x 0.6 mm in pre-operative acquisitions, GE Healthcare VCT 64). All images were denoised with the Non-local means algorithm [11], and a bias correction algorithm [12] based on intensity values was also applied on T1 MR images.

2.2 Contact Localization and Registration Workflow

Electrode contacts coordinates have to be first extracted from patient's post-operative images, and then warped into a common space to perform a retrospective study for population comparison. The spatial coordinates of each electrode contact were determined based on black artefacts from CT images, corresponding to the center of the actual contact [13]. The segmentation process included an intensity threshold, a search for the artefacts, and constraints on neighborhood. An additional step of extrapolation was necessary when just two or three contacts were identified from the four (due to the resolution of the CT scan).

We then used, as a common space, a mono-subject high-resolution 3T MRI brain template, constructed and assessed in [14]. The registration workflow was described and validated within the validation part of the template in the context of DBS in [15]: the post-operative CT was first linearly registered to the pre-operative MRI. An affine MR-to-template transformation was then computed, followed by a local affine registration computed on a region of interest within deep brain structures. With this procedure the contacts positions could be precisely warp into our template.

2.3 Clinical Scores

From numerous clinical scores assessed in our population, we studied UPDRS III (Unified PD Rating Scale [16], part III, taking into account akinesia, tremor, rigidity) widely used to assess bilateral motor improvement of patients, the Schwab & England [17] scale, and the Hoehn & Yahr [18] scale. We also studied 3 neuro-psychological scores that are often assessed through the STROOP score [19] that tests the global cognitive efficiency, and the verbal fluency tests [20] (both categorical and phonemic) that determine the ease with which patients can produce words. For each score, patients were tested without medication just before surgery (DBS OFF) and three months after it under stimulation (DBS ON). We took the difference between DBS ON and DBS OFF to compute a value that represents for all scores the degree of improvement or worsening of the patient.

2.4 Atlases

Atlases were computed as the 3D visualization of active contacts that are represented by a color code related to the patient clinical scores values. Due to errors or missing in report scoring, 15 patients were incorporated in the motor studies, and 22 in the neuro-psychological ones. Left and right contacts are shown on atlases. The x-axis represents the left-right direction, the y-axis represents the antero-posterior direction, and the z-axis represents the caudo-cranial direction.

2.5 Creation of Clusters

After atlas construction, we performed a segmentation step with the help of non-supervised techniques. The Hierarchical Ascendant Classification (HAC) was used on clinical scores and coordinates to search homogeneous groups of patients. Feature vectors are composed of 4 features: the value of the x-axis, y-axis, z-axis, and the score value: $X = (x, y, z, Score)$. The HAC operates by successively merging pairs of existing clusters, where the next pair of clusters to be merged is chosen as the pair with the smallest distance. This linkage between clusters a and b was performed with the Ward criterion along with the weighted Euclidean distance:

$$d^2(a,b) = n_a n_b \frac{\sum_{k=1}^{M} w_k (\overline{x_{ak}} - \overline{x_{bk}})}{n_a + n_b} \quad (1)$$

where $\overline{x_a} = \frac{1}{n_a} \sum_{i=1}^{n_a} x_{ai}$ is the centroid of cluster a (resp. b), n_a (resp. n_b) is the number of objects in cluster a (resp. b), and w_k are the weights, specified by $w_1 = w_2 = w_3 = \frac{1}{12}$ and $w_4 = \frac{3}{4}$. The dendrogram was cut in order to obtain two or three clusters for each clinical score. Validation of the non-supervised classification was performed with an ANOVA test. Different clusters were computed in order to correlate clinical scores and anatomical location of electrode contacts. Compare to clustering on clinical scores only, adding the coordinates permits better definition of clusters and better appreciation of the efficiency of DBS according to contacts locations.

3 Results

For all following figures, we superimposed an ellipse to improve clinical representation and interpretation. This ellipse was extracted from the segmentation of the STN by an expert, and has sensibly the same dimension of a standard STN (10 x 6 x 3 mm). For each clinical score, analyses were made for both hemispheres, but all clusters found included same patients. This assumes a symmetry of the contact coordinates between the left and the right sides of patients.

Fig. 1. shows an improvement of UPDRS III in the postero-superior region (cluster 3 in red including 2 patients), whereas the worst scores are situating mainly outside the STN and in the antero-inferior region ($p = 10^{-6}$). H&Y and S&E scores showed similar results, but with a fuzzy definition of clusters ($p = 5.10^{-2}$).

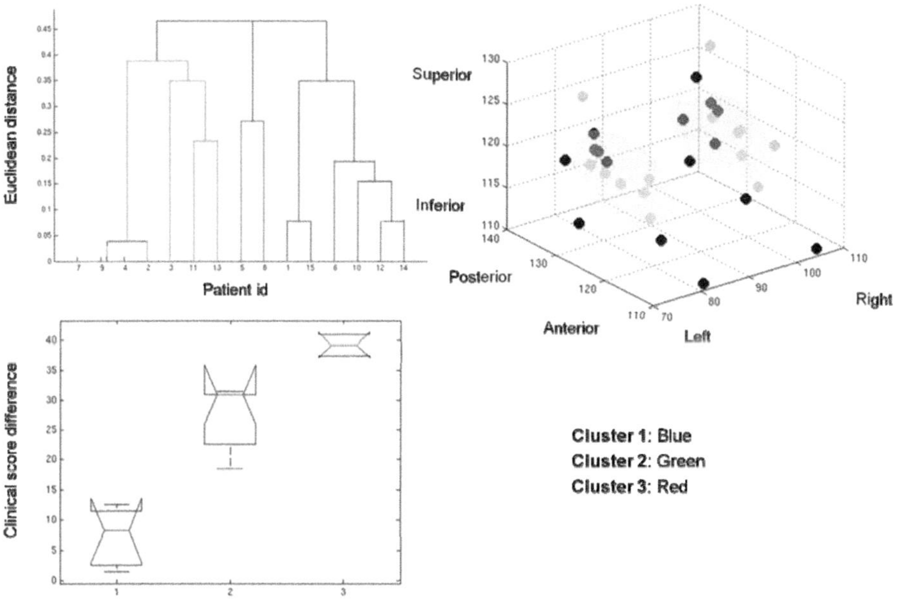

Fig. 1. UPDRS III analysis, with the dendrogram (left hemisphere), the cluster display and the ANOVA validation. Coordinates are defined in mm in the template reference space. Euclidean distances are between centroïds of clusters.

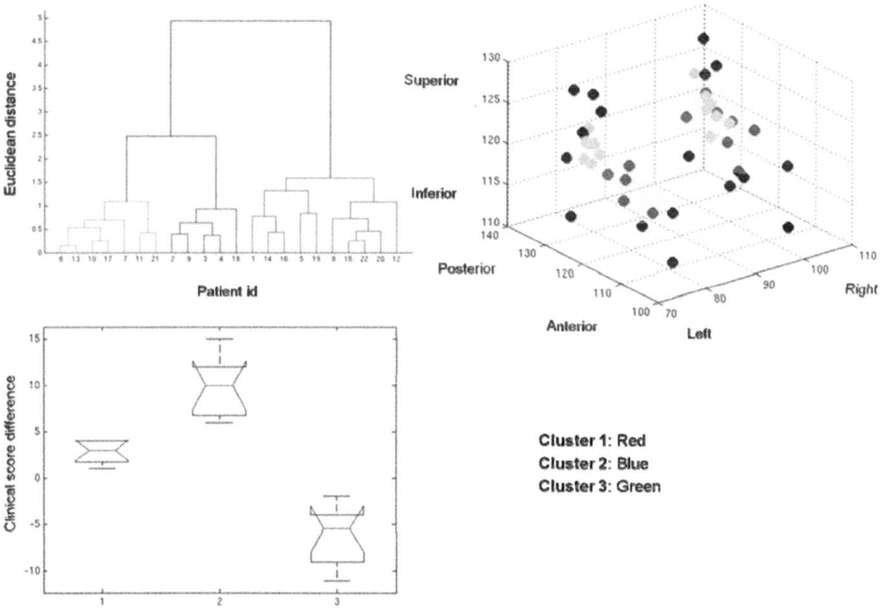

Fig. 2. Categorical fluency analysis, with the dendrogram (left side), the cluster display and the ANOVA validation. Coordinates are defined in mm in the template reference space. Euclidean distances are between centroïds of clusters.

From Fig. 2., we can see a deterioration of the categorical fluency in the posterior region (green), and an improvement in the antero region (blue) ($p = 10^{-4}$). For the phonemic fluency we found a general deterioration for all patients, without apparent separation of clusters. The analysis of the STROOP score indicated score improvement in the postero-superior region, and deterioration in the antero-inferior region ($p = 10^{-5}$).

4 Discussion

4.1 Contact Localization

Using conclusions of published works on electro-magnetic contacts effects, we have modeled the signal by a point corresponding to the center of the artifact. For further developments, it will be crucial to integrate not only the real electric current that contacts emit but also the influence of stimulation on the biological tissues. Moreover, brain shift has a real impact on the final location of electrode's contacts. A full DBS modeling would integrate all of these information to be as precise as possible.

4.2 Registration Workflow

Use of digitalized atlases is vital in DBS, for being able to help anatomical targeting. The impact of our high-resolution 3T MRI template on registration accuracy was significant and it has improved the registration quality around the basal ganglia area (about 0.8 mm. [10]). Such fusion of images should be taken with precaution, because differences of anatomy between each patient make difficult the representation of contacts in a common space. Moreover, the subject used for the mono-subject template was younger than all patients, introducing a potential bias considering the differences of anatomy between the reference subject and the patients. Nevertheless, in opposition to pure histological templates made from cadaver brain, MR templates are representing correctly in vivo anatomy of the brain.

Many active contacts are situated outside the STN within atlases. It can be partially explained by the error during the warping step, but this particularity has another explanation. First, the electrical stimulation zone is in fact larger than the simple contact position, recovering a region wide enough to accept a targeting inaccuracy. Secondly, deep brain tissues and nerves are deeply inter-connected and nerves at the periphery of structures had a role on the structure itself.

4.3 Clinical Scores

Retrospective studies with clinical data allowed understanding functional organization within deep brain structures. Each clinical score has permit to extract specific meaningful clusters. Motor scores were first analysed to assess the global outcome and then neuro-psychological scores have permitted to determine sites that were the cause of side-effects.

The main issue of this procedure is the incapacity to distinguish the response to the DBS stimulation of the right and left sided. Every test has been performed with both activated contacts. Separate evaluations would involve many hours without medication and stimulation in order to lose previous therapeutic and stimulation effects. In the preoperative targeting procedure, surgeons first localized the optimal target position of one side, and the target position of the other side was automatically computed with the definition of the midsagittal plane. These targets were used as an initial position that has to be refined per-operatively, but for this study we considered them symmetric which may explain some errors on the electrode position.

Because of their low granularity, values of the S&E and H&Y scales turned out to be less representative than UPDRS III. Even if results of motor scores studies were almost identical, the visualization of the atlas containing the UPDRS III shows that the postero-superior region was the most effective region for motor improvement. This follows conclusions of previously published works [10,21], and can be explained by the fact that this part of the STN (usually named the dorso-lateral part) is implicated in sensory and motor functions [22].

The STN is also subdivided into a ventromedial associative and a medial limbic territory. This subdivision explains that the antero-inferior (corresponding to the limbic territory) region has shown significant neuro-psychological side effects (deterioration of the Stroop score). This side effect is usually avoided by an implantation within the postero-superior region of the STN, but can easily appear if the contact is located not far from the antero-inferior region. Finally, the posterior region has shown a loss of categorical fluency. This last result was not surprising as the deterioration of the verbal fluency is one of the most observed side effects in STN DBS, with no real comprehension of the phenomena [23].

4.4 Clinical Use

The proposed anatomo-clinical atlases have been created to provide the surgeons with an additional help for better comprehension of DBS related phenomena. It could find its application in pre-operative planning as well as for post-operative assessment. As the targeting is mainly based on surgeon's knowledge and experience, it could serve as an additional source of information obtained from retrospective studies for reducing time and improving patient outcome. The underlying challenge would be to reduce the intra-operative time required for electrode's contacts adjustment by micro-electrode recordings. The actual local anaesthesia would be replaced by a general anaesthesia which would completely alter the surgical routine by reducing works of the surgical staff and improve patient's care. Alternatively, such atlases also permit to understand previous interventions which didn't give satisfactory results. In such cases, active contacts of the new patient can be warped in the common space and can be displayed.

5 Conclusion

In this paper, we focused on finding the optimum site for STN DBS by creating anatomo-clinical atlases. Such functional atlases associate anatomical position of active contacts with clinical scores for a population of cases, and are helpful for determining sites within the STN that could be the source of side effects. We showed how to extract clusters and knowledge gained from the population data based on the correlation between anatomical location of contacts and clinical data. It permits to provide the neurosurgeons with a help for targeting, but also permits to understand previous interventions which didn't give satisfactory results. This work is an example of news that can be performed in the domain, including further clinical data such as life-quality or cognitive criteria. Further studies will certainly allow learning more about DBS, better understanding of clinical side-effects and defining the optimum site for each patient according to its clinical preoperative scores.

Acknowledgments. The authors would like to acknowledge Pr. M. Vérin, Dr. S. Drapier, both neurologists from the University Hospital Of Rennes for allowing access to the clinical scores.

References

1. Benabid, A.L., Krack, P., Benazzouz, A., Limousin, P., Koudsie, A., Pollak, P.: Deep brain stimulation of the subthalamic nucleus for Parkinson's disease: methodologic aspects and clinical criteria. Neurology 55, 40–44 (2000)
2. Rodriguez-Oroz, M.C., Rodriguez, M., Guridi, J., Mewes, K., Chockkman, V., Vitek, J., DeLong, M.R., Obeso, J.A.: The subthalamic nucleus in parkinson's disease: somatotopic organization and physiological. Brain 124(9), 1777–1790 (2001)
3. Parsons, T.D., Rogers, S.A., Braayen, A.J., Woods, S.P., Troster, A.I.: Cognitive sequelae of subthalamic nucleus deep brain stimulation in Parkinson's disease: a meta-analysis. Lancet. Neurol. 5, 578–588 (2006)
4. Biseul, I., Sauleau, P., Haegelen, C., Trebon, P., Drapier, D., Raoul, S., Drapier, S., Lallement, F., Rivier, I., Lajat, Y., Verin, M.: Fear recognition is impaired by subthalamic nucleus stimulation in Parkinson's disease. Neuropsychologia 43, 1054–1059 (2005)
5. Houeto, J., Mesnage, V., Mallet, L., Pillon, B., Gargiulo, M., du Moncel, S., Bonnet, A., Pidoux, B., Dormont, D., Cornu, P., Agid, Y.: Behavioural disorders, Parkinson's disease and subthalamic stimulation. J. Neurol. Neurosurg. Psychiatry 72, 701–707 (2002)
6. St-Jean, P., Sadikot, A.F., Collins, L., Clonda, D., Kasrai, R., Evans, A.C., Peters, T.M.: Automated atlas integration and interactive three-dimensional visualization tools for planning and guidance in functional neurosurgery. IEEE Trans. on Med. Imaging 17(5), 854–866 (1998)
7. D'Haese, P.F., Cetinkaya, E., Konrad, P.E., Kao, C., Dawant, B.M.: Computer-aided placement of deep brain stimulators: From planning to intraoperative. IEEE TMI 24(11), 1469–1478 (2005)
8. D'Haese, P.F., Pallavaram, S., Li, R., Remple, M.S., Kao, C., Neimat, J.S., Konrad, P.E., Dawant, B.M.: CranialVault and its CRAVE tools: A clinical computer assistance system for deep brain stimulation (DBS) therapy. Med. Image Anal., Ahead of print (2010)
9. Guo, T., Parrent, A.G., Peters, T.M.: Surgical targeting accuracy analysis of six methods for subthalamic nucleus deep brain stimulation. Computer Aided Surgery 12(6), 325–334 (2007)
10. Pallavaram, S., Dawant, B.M., Remple, M., Neimat, J.S., Kao, C., Konrad, P.E., D'Haese, P.F.: Effect of brain shift on the creation of functional atlases for deep brain stimulation surgery. Int. J. Comp. Assist Radiol. Surg. 5(3), 221–228 (2009)
11. Coupe P, Yger P, Prima S, Hellier P, Kervrann C, Barillot C. An Optimized Blockwise Non Local Means Denoising Filter for 3D Magnetic Resonance Images. IEEE TMI 24(4), 425-441 (2008)

12. Mangin, J.F.: Entropy minimization for automatic correction of intensity non uniformity. In: Proc. of the IEEE Workshop on Math. Method in Biomed. Image Analysis, MMBIA 2000, Hilton Head Island, pp. 162–169 (2000)
13. Pollo, C., Villemure, J.G., Vingerhoets, F., Ghika, J., Maeder, P., Meuli, R.: Magnetic resonance artefact induced by the electrode activa 3389: an in vitro and in vivo study. Acta Neurochirurgica 146(2), 161–164 (2004)
14. Lalys, F., Haegelen, C., Ferre, J.C., El-Ganaoui, O., Jannin, P.: Construction and assessment of a 3T MRI brain template. NeuroImage 49, 345–354 (2010)
15. Lalys, F., Haegelen, C., Abadie, A., Jannin, P.: Post-operative assessment in Deep Brain Stimulation based on multimodal images: registration workow and validation. In: Proceedings of SPIE, vol. 7261 (2009)
16. Fahn, Y., Elton, R.: Unified Parkinson's disease rating scale. In: Fahn, S., Marsden, C., Calne, D., Goldstein, M. (eds.) Recent Developments in Parkinson's Disease, vol. 2, pp. 153–163. Macmillan, Florham Park (1987)
17. Schwab, R.S., England Jr., A.: Projection techniques for evaluating surgery in Parkinson's Disease, pp. 152–157 (1968)
18. Hoehn, M., Yahr, M.: Parkinsonism: onset, progression and mortality. Neurology 17(5), 427–442 (1967)
19. Stroop, J.R.: Studies of interference in serial verbal reactions. Journal of Experimental Psychology 18, 643–661 (1935)
20. Troyer, A.K., Moscovitch, M., Winocur, G., Leach, L., Freedman, M.: Clustering and switching on verbal fluency tests in Alzheimer's and Parkinson's disease. J. Int. Neuropsycholog. Soc. 4(2), 137–143 (1998)
21. Lanotte, M.M., Rizzone, M., Bergamasco, B., Faccani, G., Melcarne, A., Lopiano, L.: Deep Brain Stimulation of the subthalamic nucleus: anatomical, neurophysiological, and outcome correlations with the effects of stimulation. J. Neurol Neurosurg. Psychiatry 72, 53–58 (2002)
22. Theodosopoulos, P.V., Marks, W.J., Christine, C., Starr, P.A.: Locations of movement-related cells in the human subthalamic nucleus in parkinson's disease. Movement Disorders 18(7), 791–798 (2003)
23. Saint-Cyr, J.A., Trépanier, L.L., Kumar, R., Lozano, A.M., Lang, A.E.: Neuropsychological consequences of chronic stimulation of the subthalamic nucleus in Parkinson's disease. Brain 123, 2091–2108 (2000)

Intra-operative "Pick-Up" Ultrasound for Robot Assisted Surgery with Vessel Extraction and Registration: A Feasibility Study

Caitlin Schneider[1], Julian Guerrero[1], Christopher Nguan[2], Robert Rohling[1], and Septimiu Salcudean[1]

[1] Electrical and Computer Engineering, University of British Columbia
[2] Department of Urology, Vancouver General Hospital

Abstract. We propose the use of a "pick-up" ultrasound transducer for robot-assisted minimally invasive surgeries. Unlike prior approaches, the ultrasound transducer is inserted before the procedure and remains in the abdominal cavity throughout. We present a new design for such an intra-abdominal ultrasound transducer with a handle that can be grasped in a repeatable manner using a da Vinci Pro-Grasp tool. The main application is mapping the vasculature, which is segmented from Doppler and B-mode images using a Kalman-filtering approach. Our goal is employ the vasculature to register pre-operative CT to intra-operative camera images. To demonstrate the feasibility of the approach, we use an ultrasound flow phantom to register a CT surface model to extracted ultrasound vessel center points using an iterative closest point method. The transducer was tracked with electromagnetic sensors and a target registration error of 3.2 mm was calculated. The initial application will be nephrectomy where vessel localization is paramount.

Keywords: Robotic surgery, kidney, ultrasound, CT, image registration.

1 Introduction

Laparoscopic partial and radical nephrectomy requires that the renal artery and vein be located before the resection can begin. Because approximately 25% of cardiac output, or about 1.5 L/min, flows through the kidneys, and because the surgeon is working in close proximity to the patient's aorta and vena cava, caution must be used during the dissection in order to avoid damaging these major vessels. Knowledge of the vessels' location during the procedure would provide surgeons with information to complete a safe and precise dissection. By providing this information, it is expected that the surgeon's confidence will increase and the dissection time required to mobilize the kidney will decrease from the current time of 1-1.5 hours at our center, where an average of ten to fifteen procedures are completed per year.

Robotic technology, such as the da Vinci Surgical System (Intuitive Surgical Inc, Sunnyvale, CA), is increasingly used in a variety of surgical procedures. The da Vinci system attempts to improve the techniques of laparoscopic surgery

R.H. Taylor and G.-Z. Yang (Eds.): IPCAI 2011, LNCS 6689, pp. 122–132, 2011.

through the dexterity of the tools and quality of the stereoscopic cameras. The system allows surgeons to work in a manner that mimics open surgery but has the benefits of small laparoscopic incisions. Due to its stereoscopic display, the robot system provides a platform to include image guidance, which could improve patient outcomes and decrease surgery time.

Traditional laparoscopic intra-abdominal ultrasound (IAUS) is currently used for a variety of procedures, including resection of liver cancer [1], gall bladder removal [3] and resection of kidney cancer [12]. IAUS provides high-quality real-time intra-operative imaging for assessment of tumour margins, guidance around vessels and locating tumour resection planes.

Although traditional laparoscopic ultrasound instruments are valuable imaging tools in many types of surgery, they have limited mobility. During robotic laparoscopic surgery, they are typically controlled by the patient-side assistant instead of the operating surgeon. While in use, the IAUS transducer requires a dedicated port. Therefore, each time the transducer is needed, a tool change must take place. An ultrasound transducer that is controlled by the da Vinci masters and modeled after a typical da Vinci 5-mm tool has been proposed previously [14]. However, this tool still requires dedicated port or tool changes, and is limited in its orientation by the tool wrist.

A significant application of intra-operative ultrasound is the localization of vessels in the surgical field. Localized vessels can be used to define surgical planes and to register intra-operative images to pre-operative scans. Vessels have been previously used to register intra-operative data to pre-operative CT and magnetic resonance imaging (MRI) scans [8,10,11,7,13]. For example, the cortical vessels of the brain can orient the surgeon and account for brain deformation during image guided surgery through video tracking of the vessels [10] or tracked ultrasound [13]. Image guidance during liver surgery is another application in which vessels are used for registration [8,11] because the vessels of the liver are prominent features in surgical navigation for tumour resection. Previous methods have involved voxel-based registration [11], image-to-model registration [7] and model-to-model registration [13,8]. Model-to-model registration methods typically use a modified version of the iterative closest point (ICP) algorithm [2] applied to the vessel centerlines. Other methods use Doppler images to create a model from the US images with region growing segmentation [8] or color-based segmentation [13]. This paper presents an algorithm that will have both the centerlines of the vessel tree and the surface model as inputs to an ICP-based registration.

In this paper, a new custom-built ultrasound transducer that offers greater flexibility is described, and its use in intra-operative imaging and registration to pre-operative imaging is demonstrated. The primary application discussed is robot-assisted partial nephrectomy. This paper also describes and examines an automatic method of initializing, segmenting and registering vessels. Using a combination of power Doppler and B-mode ultrasound, vessel contours are found, and through the use of a tracked transducer, the 2D contours are combined to create a 3D model of the renal vessels and branches. The centerline representation of the vessel contours is then registered to pre-operative CT using an ICP algorithm.

2 Materials and Methods

Intra-Abdominal Transducer Design. In order to take advantage of the degrees of freedom (DOF) available with the da Vinci wristed tools, a new intra-abdominal pick-up transducer was designed to fulfill the following design parameters [Figure 1]. The design requirements for this new transducer were determined through consultations with the surgeons at our center and a transducer manufacturer. The completed transducer will be small enough to fit through a standard laparoscopic incision and be maneuverable within the abdominal cavity. The da Vinci tools will be able to grasp the transducer in a repeatable manner and create a fixed transformation between the tool location and the ultrasound image, i.e. the transducer's motion should also be fully constrained once grasped. Finally, the tool should self-align with a 'locking' mechanism on the transducer, such that the tool and transducer need not be initially well aligned to guarantee capture.

The transducer will be placed into the abdominal cavity before the laparoscopic cannulas. The transducer tether will pass alongside the camera cannula, but through the same skin incision. Thus, ultrasound imaging is available throughout the operation, without the need for tool changes. This minimizes the effect of using the transducer on surgical workflow. When the probe is not in use, it will stay within the abdomen on a long tether, which will limit the stress on the patient's incision.

A hardened steel section, the lap-handle, was added to the transducer to allow for non-damaging, repetitive tool grasping [Figure 1,2]. Grasping at the proximal end also reduces the risk of damage to the transducer face. The lap-handle features a wide groove and two pins. Since the transducer must be grasped quickly, it has been designed to have a self-aligning grasp. Sloped sides of the groove allow for a wider capture range, while a short wall on one side ensures that the transducer is always grasped repeatably and securely with respect to

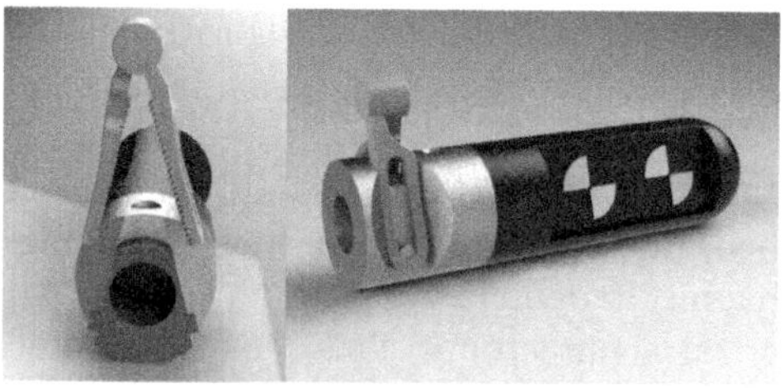

Fig. 1. Rendered images of the IAUS transducer. Left: cross sectional view (blue) of the lap-handle, a steel section added to the transducer. The angled faces and locking pins can be seen. Right: the tool fits tightly against the angled faces. The practicality of adding visual tracking markers is demonstrated.

the robot tool. The pins fit within the slot of the da Vinci Pro-Grasp Forceps (model 420093) and constrain all 6 degrees of freedom of the probe.

In addition to the lap-handle at the transducer's proximal end, the transducer shape also contributes to its versatility. Two faces have been cut into the sides of the transducer at an angle similar to that of da Vinci and laparoscopic tool jaws. These faces allow for additional flanges to be snapped over the top of the transducer. The flanges could include ways for other da Vinci or standard laparoscopic tools to grasp the transducer (different tools and different angles) or specialized markers to aid in vision-based tracking [Figure 1]. An electromagnetic (EM) position and orientation sensor (Ascension Technologies, Burlington, VT) is also embedded in the transducer to aid in transducer tracking. The transducer and sensor cables are integrated into the housing design to allow standard surgical sterilization protocols to be followed.

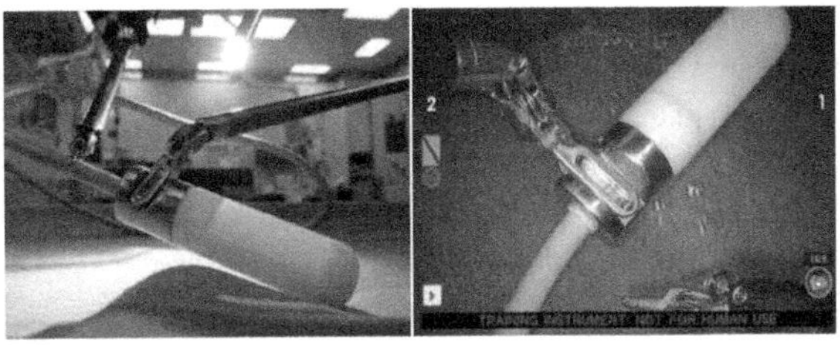

Fig. 2. The pick-up IAUS transducer is grasped and manipulated by the Pro-Grasp tool of the da Vinci Surgical System

Image Processing and Registration. A method has previously been developed to segment and create a 3D vessel model from ultrasound, using the combined vessel wall detection in B-mode images and the Doppler flow signal [5]. A centerline representation will be created from the contour-based model.

Since the vessel identification has to be carried out during surgery when user interaction with software should be minimized, the power Doppler signal is used to initialize and guide the vessel segmentation in B-mode images. This enables multiple vessels to be segmented simultaneously and automatically. Doppler provides high contrast for vessels with high flow, but is susceptible to motion artifacts. On the other hand, B-mode segmentation relies on the difference in echogenicity of the vessels compared with surrounding tissue. As the kidney vessels branch and enter the kidney, distinctive boundaries are no longer visible. Thus it is best to combine the two modalities to create reliable vessel segmentations.

To create the contours of the vessels, a modified Star-Kalman filter predicts vessel contours in each ultrasound image. The predicted shape is assumed to be elliptical, although the vessels can deviate from the elliptical shape when strong edges are present without affecting the performance of the algorithm. A temporal Kalman filter is used to track the vessel center across frames. Gradients in the B-mode image are used to find the vessel walls. An interacting multiple model (IMM) system is implemented to combine data from B-mode and Doppler images as well as previously created contours [5]. The transformation between the US image and the sensor is known from prior calibration, and thus the centroid of each contour is found in the sensor base-unit coordinate system. The Doppler signal can define the original seed point for the Star-Kalman algorithm to minimize the need for user interaction.

After the US vessels are segmented, the contour centroids from each 2D slice became the targets for registration to the CT model. In our approach, we have started with a rigid-body ICP algorithm that was used to align the CT surface with the sparse US representation. The Visual Toolkit implementation of ICP was used; it employs points, lines and surfaces in its calculations of closest points. The CT is the source for the registration such that the errors between the surface and the US points are minimized when the US points are centered within the CT vessels.

User initialization is needed to place the source and target within the capture range of the registration algorithm. Robotic surgery for the kidney has a very predictable set-up, in which the robot is positioned behind the patient, who is placed in the flank position, and the ultrasound machine (and EM transmitter) will be next to the robot and towards the patients head. The expected orientation of the patient with respect to the EM transmitter can be calculated before the initial US images are taken, and the approximate initial transformation between the two coordinate frames can be determined.

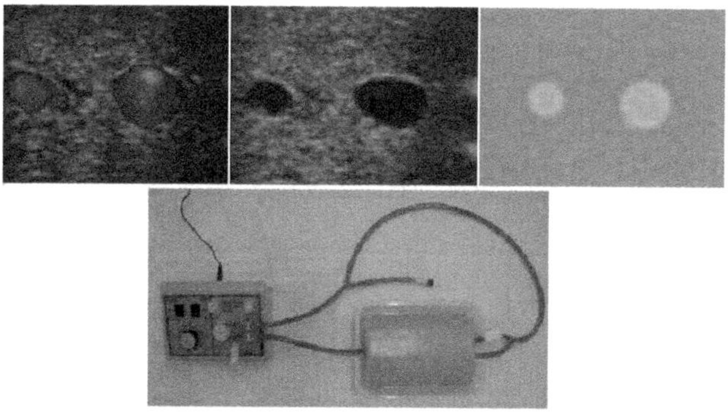

Fig. 3. The ultrasound flow phantom used for these studies. Top Left: power Doppler, top middle: B-mode images and top right: CT imaging, bottom: photograph of the phantom.

Experimental Setup and Data Anaylsis. In order to gain insight in to the properties of the kidney vessels, ultrasound images were taken from several patients with a traditional laparoscopic ultrasound transducer during radical nephrectomy. Images of both the internal vasculature and renal vessels were recorded. All imaging was performed with default vascular parameters by a surgeon not specialized in ultrasonography, using a traditional IAUS transducer and machine (Philips HDI 5000, Philips Healthcare, Andover, MA).

For feasibility testing of the registration method, a combination of components including an US machine, an EM tracker and the associated data and image processing software was used. A PC-based Ultrasonix RP ultrasound machine with a research interface (Ultrasonix Corp, Richmond, BC) allowed for access to the imaging stream and the imaging parameters during testing. This interface allowed for separate B-mode and power Doppler images to be directly streamed. For all phantom work, a linear 10MHz vascular transducer (L12-5) was used. This transducer array has 128 elements and is approximately 3.8cm in length. A miniBird sensor (Ascension Technologies) was rigidly attached to the transducer. The resolution of the sensor is specified as 0.5 mm and 0.1 degrees for positions and orientation with an accuracy of 1.8 mm and 0.5 degrees, respectively. A z-wire calibration [9] was used to find the homogeneous transformation between the sensor and the ultrasound image. All processing was completed using the on-board computer of the ultrasound machine.

A custom designed flow phantom (Blue Phantom, Redmond, WA) was constructed and used in validation experiments. This phantom consists of a single vessel that branches once midway through the phantom. The internal vessel diameter varies from 4 to 6 mm. A peristaltic pump mimics the flow profile of blood flowing through arteries. Cross-sections and overall images of the phantom are shown in Figure 3.

A CT scan of this phantom was taken with 0.3-mm isoptropic resolution. The vessels were segmented manually from the CT scan, and a 3D surface model was constructed [16]. Model correspondence with each CT slice was checked visually. Eighteen 2-mm steel spheres were secured under the phantom and served as visual fiducial landmarks in both the CT and US to quantify the error in registration. The vector displacements from the final transformed fiducial landmarks in US to the corresponding CT landmarks were used to quantify the target registration error (TRE). These fiducials were manually segmented in the ultrasound images during vessel segmentation. Similar spheres at the air-tissue interface have been employed for fidicial registration [18]. The repeatability of identifying the fiducial locations, or fiducial localization error, was tested in the ultrasound images of this phantom. For each of five different fiducials, the fiducial locations were identified in ten images taken at a variety of angles. The centroid of each

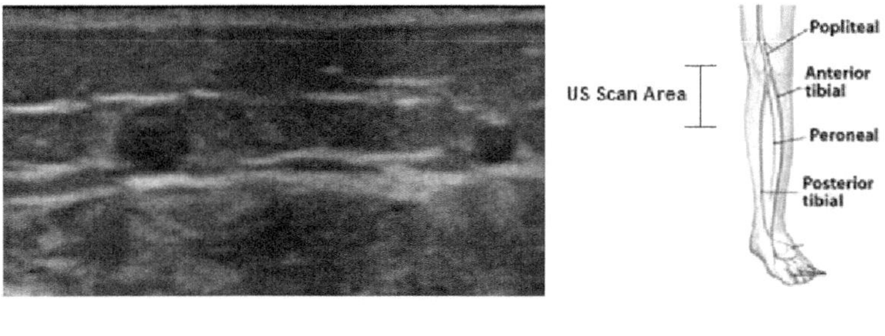

Fig. 4. Left: example ultrasound image of the leg. Right: schmatic drawing of the US scan area.

grouping was found and the displacement from the centroid to each point, the target localization error, was calculated to estimate the point cloud distribution.

Twelve US models of the phantom, consisting of vessel centroids, were created through the contour-based Kalman filtering algorithm during the US scans. The CT segmented surface model and the US centerlines were then registered through the ICP algorithm described above.

In order to validate this segmentation algorithm *in vivo*, the algorithm was tested using the anterior and posterior tibial arteries and the popliteal artery [Figure 4]. These vessels were scanned around the branching point to simulate the branching of the renal artery. A surface model of the vessels was created using manual segmentation of a 3D ultrasound scan created with Stradwin [16]. 3D ultrasound was used instead of CT to avoid the volunteer's exposure to radiation. The vessels were scanned a second time and segmented in real time using the contour-based Kalman filtering algorithm described above. Branching points in the vessel structures were used as target registration points. An example US image of the vessels and scan area can be seen in Figure 4.

Overall, three sets of experiments were completed. First, to determine the feasibility of using Power Doppler for vessel segmentation during kidney surgery, preliminary IAUS data from patients undergoing kidney surgery was collected. Next, the registration algorithm was validated through phantom studies. Finally, an *in vivo* registration was tested on the anterior and posterior tibial arteries and the popliteal artery.

3 Results

In the first set of experiments, IAUS images were collected from five patients undergoing radical nephrectomy. Sample ultrasound images of the kidney taken from a laparoscopic transducer highlight the high-quality that is available with this method, and the ease of vessel detection using Doppler methods [Figure 5].

During the phantom studies, a series of twelve vessel models of the ultrasound phantom were created during separate US scans using the Kalman filtering algorithm. These models were registered to the CT [Figure 6]. The target registration error was found based on an average of 10 fiducials per model. The RMS error for all landmarks was 3.2 mm. The distribution of these target registration errors

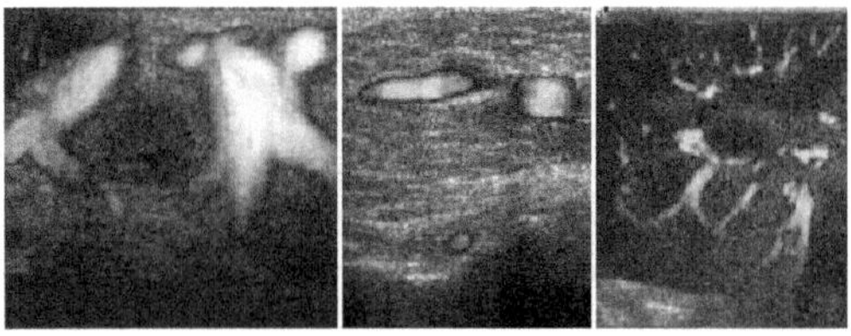

Fig. 5. Example images for intra-operative power Doppler images of the kidney vessels. Left: Branching of renal artery. Middle: renal artery and vein. Right: internal vessels of the kidney.

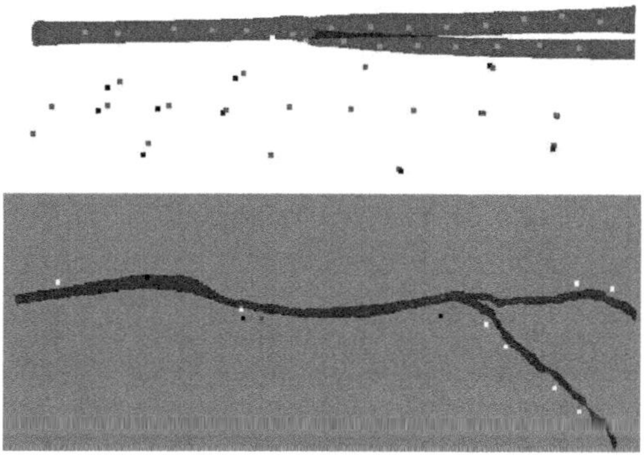

Fig. 6. Top: Example of the completed registration. The blue surface model represents the CT model of the vessel phantom, and the red points are the fiducial locations. The series of the white points represent the ultrasound contour centroids, paired with the black fiducial points. Bottom: Final registration of the anterior and posterior tibial arteries and the popliteal artery. The surface model was created from 3D ultrasound.

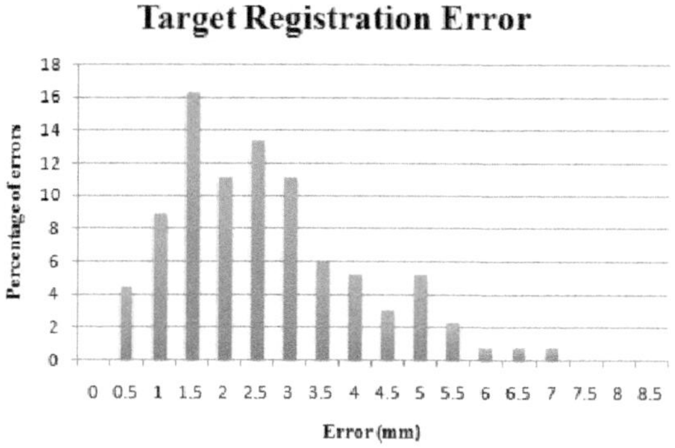

Fig. 7. Distribution of registration errors for a series of 12 CT to ultrasound vessel registrations using the vessel phantom

(TRE) ranged from 0.73 to 7.07 mm [Figure 7]. The average error along each axis was also found, in which the x-axis is in the direction of flow through the vessels and the y-axis is in plane with the vessel branch. The average error for all fiducials was 1.9 ± 1.7 mm, 1.3 ± 0.4 mm and 1.04 ± 0.41 mm, for the x, y and z directions respectively. As part of the experiment, the fiducial localization error was also found from the ultrasound images. The RMS error for fiducial localization was 0.83 mm.

During the registration of *in vivo* vessels, 7 scans were taken of the anterior and posterior tibial arteries and the popliteal artery [Figure 6]. Registration landmarks were chosen at two small branching points and the main branch point within the vessel structure. An RMS error of 7.5 mm was calculated using these targets.

4 Discussion

The new pick-up ultrasound concept has been successfully tested with the da Vinci robot. The lap-handle allows the transducer to be easily grasped and provides the transducer with the same freedom of motion as the da Vinci tools (see video). The transducer could be easily grasped by the da Vinci tools due to its self-aligning properties. During testing, the capture range was found to be approximately 20 degrees from each axis of the transducer.

Our goal is to provide the surgeon additional image guidance through the stereo camera display of the da Vinci robot. In order for this to be possible, the location of the transducer must be known in the coordinate frame of the camera. There are several ways in which the transducer location may be tracked. Due to the repeatability of the tool/transducer transformation, the joint angles of the da Vinci tool can determine the transducer's position and orientation, and thus the US image plane location. Similar pose determination methods applied to the camera combined with camera calibration allows the ultrasound image to be transformed into camera coordinates and displayed in the surgeon's stereo console. EM tracking provides an alternative method and the transducer includes a 6DOF EM tracker. EM trackers are small, unobtrusive, and do not require additional large pieces of equipment in the operating room. High accuracies have been reported in the range of 1% of the dimension of interest [6] and have been tested in clinical environments [17]. A third method of tracking is purely vision based [4]. Using the da Vinci stereo cameras, the transducer can be tracked using purely image processing techniques such as feature tracking and the disparity between the stereo camera images. This allows direct transformation from the ultrasound image to camera coordinates.

The registrations between US centroids in our phantom and CT model had a TRE of 3.2 mm. The errors between fiducials in the two modalities were within the range of what has been reported previously, with errors ranging from 1.3 mm to 5 mm for deformable and rigid registrations [10,8,11]. The errors calculated along each axis demonstrate that the x-axis has the greatest overall error, 1.9 ± 1.7 mm. Due to the low angle of the branch (only a few degrees), and the fact that there is only a single branch, the registration in this direction is not as well defined as the other directions. In a real vessel structure that has more branches and greater diversity in vessel directions and shape, such as seen in the vessels entering the kidney, the registration would be more constrained, and the errors expected to be smaller. The 0.83 mm error in the fiducial localization accounts for a small amount of the overall registration errors. An RMS error of 7.5 mm was calculated during the *in vivo* studies, Similar to the phantom studies, this vessel system had a single narrow angle branch which does not completely constrain the registration along the long axis. The targets used for this registration may have also contributed to the error. Branch points were chosen as recognizable features, but the exact location of the branching is not always well defined. In addition, patient motion and changes in vessel location due to probe pressure may have contributed to the registration errors.

In a clinical setting, additional sources of error may be present. Some errors due to organ motion are expected, caused by changes in the patient position and insufflation. These errors will be explored further during patient testing. It is hoped that the strong attachment of the kidney and aorta to the patients' thoracic walls will limit the motion due to patient position. Organ deformation during the procedure may cause the internal organs to shift as well, which will result in some error in a rigid registration. Errors from patient position may be present, but can be accounted for using flank preoperative CT scans. Deformation due to insufflation will be determined during the studies and could possibly be predicted through patient specific modeling. We envision that the CT registration will be used during the first stages of surgery before major deformation during the procedure has occurred. This will allow the surgeon to use the CT for general navigation and initial kidney and tumor localization. Later in the surgical procedure, the probe can be used to locally view and create models of the vessels.

5 Conclusion and Future Work

A system for integration of pick-up intra-abdominal ultrasound into robotic surgery has been proposed and initial feasibility tests completed. With a new ultrasound transducer, IAUS is feasible throughout the duration of the procedure. The transducer can be sterilized and has provisions for expanded usability with other laparoscopic tools. The vessels of the kidney are quite distinct in ultrasound and their high flow allows high quality Doppler ultrasound images to be created.

We propose the use of ultrasound to CT registration for the initial stages of dissection, to give the surgeon a better sense of orientation and direction. This is even more important for surgeons inexperienced with the da Vinci robot.

Future work will include patient trials with the new transducer to assess its usability and functionality. Using the pre-operative CT, the best method of presenting the registered CT to the surgeon will be determined. Augmented reality, through different types of overlay, has had positive results [15]. A similar system will be implemented using our new 'pick-up' ultrasound concept, and targeted at highlighting the renal and surrounding vessels since these are important targets for dissection.

References

1. Barbot, D.J.: Improved staging of liver tumors using laparscopic intraoperative ultrasound. Journal of Surgical Oncology 64, 63–67 (1997)
2. Besl, P., McKay, N.: A method for registration of 3-D shapes. IEEE Transactions on Pattern Analysis and Machine Intelligence, 239–256 (1992)
3. Catheline, J.M.: A comparison of laparoscopic ultrasound versus cholangiography in the evaluation of the biliary tree during laparoscopic cholecystectomy. European Journal of Ultrasound 10(1), 1–9 (1999)

4. Dutkiewicz, P., Kietczewski, M., Kowalski, M., Wroblewski, W.: Experimental verification of visual tracking of surgical tools. In: Robot Motion and Control, pp. 237–242. IEEE, Los Alamitos (2005)
5. Guerrero, J., Salcudean, S., McEwen, J., Masri, B., Nicolaou, S.: Real-time vessel segmentation and tracking for ultrasound imaging applications. IEEE Transactions on Medical Imaging 26(8), 1079–1090 (2007)
6. Hughes, S., D'Arcy, T., Maxwell, D., Chiu, W., Milner, A., Saunders, J., Sheppard, R.: Volume estimation from multiplanar 2D ultrasound images using a remote electromagnetic position and orientation sensor. Ultrasound in Medicine & Biology 22(5), 561–572 (1996)
7. Jomier, J., Aylward, S.R.: Rigid and deformable vasculature-to-image registration: A hierarchical approach. In: Barillot, C., Haynor, D.R., Hellier, P. (eds.) MICCAI 2004. LNCS, vol. 3216, pp. 829–836. Springer, Heidelberg (2004)
8. Lange, T., Eulenstein, S., Huenerbein, M., Lamecker, H., Schlag, P.: Augmenting intraoperative 3D ultrasound with preoperative models for navigation in liver surgery. In: Barillot, C., Haynor, D.R., Hellier, P. (eds.) MICCAI 2004. LNCS, vol. 3217, pp. 534–541. Springer, Heidelberg (2004)
9. Mercier, L., Langø, T., Lindseth, F., Collins, L.: A review of calibration techniques for freehand 3-D ultrasound systems. Ultrasound in Medicine & Biology 31(2), 143–165 (2005)
10. Nakajima, S., Atsumi, H., Kikinis, R., Moriarty, T., Metcalf, D., Jolesz, F., Black, P.: Use of cortical surface vessel registration for image-guided neurosurgery. Neurosurgery 40(6), 1201 (1997)
11. Penney, G., Blackall, J., Hamady, M., Sabharwal, T., Adam, A., Hawkes, D.: Registration of freehand 3D ultrasound and magnetic resonance liver images. Medical Image Analysis 8(1), 81–91 (2004)
12. Polascik, T., Meng, M., Epstein, J., Marshall, F.: Intraoperative sonography for the evaluation and management of renal tumors: Experience with 100 patients. The Journal of Urology 154(5), 1676–1680 (1995)
13. Reinertsen, I., Descoteaux, M., Siddiqi, K., Collins, D.: Validation of vessel-based registration for correction of brain shift. Medical Image Analysis 11(4), 374–388 (2007)
14. Schneider, C., Dachs, G., Hasser, C., Choti, M., DiMaio, S., Taylor, R.: Robot-assisted laparoscopic ultrasound. In: Information Processing in Computer-Assisted Interventions, pp. 67–80 (2010)
15. Su, L., Vagvolgyi, B., Agarwal, R., Reiley, C., Taylor, R., Hager, G.: Augmented reality during robot-assisted laparoscopic partial nephrectomy: Toward real-time 3D-CT to stereoscopic video registration. Urology 73(4), 896–900 (2009)
16. Treece, G., Prager, R., Gee, A.: Regularised marching tetrahedra: improved iso-surface extraction. Computers & Graphics 23(4), 583–598 (1999)
17. Yaniv, Z., Wilson, E., Lindisch, D., Cleary, K.: Electromagnetic tracking in the clinical environment. Medical Physics 36, 876 (2009)
18. Yip, M.C., Adebar, T.K., Rohling, R.N., Salcudean, S.E., Nguan, C.Y.: 3D ultrasound to stereoscopic camera registration through an air-tissue boundary. In: Jiang, T., Navab, N., Pluim, J.P.W., Viergever, M.A. (eds.) MICCAI 2010. LNCS, vol. 6362, pp. 626–634. Springer, Heidelberg (2010)

Constrained 2-D/3-D Registration for Motion Compensation in AFib Ablation Procedures

Alexander Brost[1,*], Andreas Wimmer[1], Rui Liao[2], Joachim Hornegger[1], and Norbert Strobel[3]

[1] Pattern Recognition Lab, Friedrich-Alexander-University Erlangen-Nuremberg, Erlangen, Germany
Alexander.Brost@informatik.uni-erlangen.de
[2] Siemens Corporate Research, Imaging and Visualization, Princeton, NJ, USA
[3] Siemens AG, Healthcare, Forchheim, Germany

Abstract. Fluoroscopic overlay images rendered from pre-operative volumetric data can provide additional guidance for physicians during catheter ablation procedures for treatment of atrial fibrillation (AFib). As these overlay images are compromised by cardiac and respiratory motion, motion compensation methods have been proposed. The approaches so far either require simultaneous biplane imaging for 3-D motion compensation or, in case of mono-plane X-ray imaging, provide only a limited 2-D functionality. To overcome the downsides of the previously suggested methods, we propose a new approach that facilitates full 3-D motion compensation even if only mono-plane X-ray views are available. To this end, we use constrained model-based 2-D/3-D registration to track a circumferential mapping catheter which is commonly used during AFib catheter ablation procedures. Our approach yields an average 2-D tracking error of 0.6 mm and an average 3-D tracking error of 2.1 mm.

1 Introduction

Atrial fibrillation (AFib), which is the most common arrhythmia, leads to an increased risk of stroke for the patient [1]. After the first treatment approaches using radio-frequency ablations by Haïssaguerre et al. [2], this method has now become an accepted treatment option [3]. Catheter ablation procedures are performed in electrophysiology (EP) labs usually equipped with modern C-arm X-ray systems. These devices often provide 3-D imaging of the heart [4] to overcome the issue that soft-tissue of the heard is difficult to see in X-ray images. Electro-anatomic mapping systems have been proposed in the past to show the catheter position in 3-D within a registered pre-operative data set [5,6,7,8]. While they promise to save X-ray dose, they add effort and cost to the procedure. In addition, mapping systems are virtual reality systems. They do not allow to instantly confirm catheter positions under X-ray with respect to detailed 3-D cardiac anatomy. In some instances, they may even be off with respect to the

* Corresponding author.

R.H. Taylor and G.-Z. Yang (Eds.): IPCAI 2011, LNCS 6689, pp. 133–144, 2011.

underlying anatomy [9]. Augmented fluoroscopy, using either CT, MRI or C-arm CT, overlaying a pre-operative data set onto live fluoroscopic images can facilitate more precise catheter navigation and also reduce fluoroscopy time [10,11,12]. Unfortunately, catheter navigation under augmented fluoroscopy is compromised by cardiac and respiratory motion. A first approach to overcome this problem by providing a motion compensated overlay has been proposed in [13]. It involved tracking of commonly used circumferential mapping catheters. As atrial fibrillation (Afib) therapy takes place in the vicinity of the circumferential mapping catheter, catheter tracking can be assumed to capture the motion of the relevant treatment region correctly if the device has been firmly positioned. Fortunately, we can count on the physicians to provide us with a stable wall contact, as it is in their best interest. Otherwise complete isolation of the pulmonary veins (PVs) may fail due to undetected residual PV-atrial electrical connections. The intial proposed method generates a 3-D model of the catheter and applies an unconstrained 2-D/3-D registration to register the catheter model to biplane fluoroscopy images. In the first approach, a filter-based technique using a vessel enhancement filtering was used. The method was later extended by integrating a learning-based catheter segmentation [14]. However, this technique still required simultaneous biplane imaging. An approach for monoplane fluoroscopic imaging was introduced in [15] considering only a 2-D catheter and moving the overlay. That is, the projection of the pre-operative 3-D data set is shifted on the live fluoroscopic images in sync with the cardiac and respiratory motion. The last method might be the approach of choice if only a monoplane C-arm system is available. In EP labs equipped with biplane C-arm systems, often only one imaging plane is used at a time to reduce the dose to the patient. In this case, the methods suggested in [13,14] are not applicable. The 2-D method described in [15] is not ideal either, as it requires re-initialization of the catheter model as soon as the C-arm view direction changes. To improve the mono-plane situation, we propose a constrained 2-D/3-D registration to perform motion compensation using a 3-D catheter model. The generation of a 3-D catheter model requires only a single biplane shot. This way, the increase of X-ray radiation to the patient is kept to a minimum.

2 Three-Dimensional Catheter Model

In the first step of our method, a 3-D model of the circumferential mapping catheter is generated, as proposed in [13,16,14]. A single biplane frame is required to manually initialize the model generation step. Therefore, 2-D points $\boldsymbol{p}_{\mathrm{A}}, \boldsymbol{p}_{\mathrm{B}} \in \mathbb{R}^2$ are selected on the elliptically shaped part of the catheter in each imaging plane. The imaging planes are denoted by A and B. Two-dimensional ellipses $\boldsymbol{C}_{\mathrm{A}}, \boldsymbol{C}_{\mathrm{B}} \in \mathbb{R}^{3\times 3}$ are then fitted to these points. These matrices fulfill the following equations

$$\boldsymbol{p}_{\mathrm{A}}^T \boldsymbol{C}_{\mathrm{A}} \boldsymbol{p}_{\mathrm{A}} = 0 \quad (1)$$

$$\boldsymbol{p}_{\mathrm{B}}^T \boldsymbol{C}_{\mathrm{B}} \boldsymbol{p}_{\mathrm{B}} = 0. \quad (2)$$

Two 3-D cones $\boldsymbol{Q}_{\mathrm{A}}, \boldsymbol{Q}_{\mathrm{B}} \in \mathbb{R}^{4\times 4}$ are then computed by using the projection matrices $\boldsymbol{P}_{\mathrm{A}}, \boldsymbol{P}_{\mathrm{B}} \in \mathbb{R}^{3\times 4}$

$$\boldsymbol{Q}_{\mathrm{A}} = \boldsymbol{P}_{\mathrm{A}}^T \boldsymbol{C}_{\mathrm{A}} \boldsymbol{P}_{\mathrm{A}} \tag{3}$$

$$\boldsymbol{Q}_{\mathrm{B}} = \boldsymbol{P}_{\mathrm{B}}^T \boldsymbol{C}_{\mathrm{B}} \boldsymbol{P}_{\mathrm{B}}. \tag{4}$$

These two 3-D cones are defined by the position of the X-ray tube relative to the projection of the elliptical catheter onto the imaging plane. The 3-D catheter model is computed by intersecting the two elliptical cones $\boldsymbol{Q}_A$ and $\boldsymbol{Q}_B$ corresponding to plane A and plane B of a biplane system respectively [17]. The solution is found by calculating η such that the quadric

$$\boldsymbol{Q}(\eta) = \boldsymbol{Q}_A + \eta \boldsymbol{Q}_B \tag{5}$$

is of rank 2 [17]. As pointed out in [13], there are two possible solutions. Prior knowledge about the pseudo-circular shape of the mapping catheter is used and the result that is more circular is chosen. The simulation results in [16] verify this assumption. The 3-D model is denoted as $\boldsymbol{m}_i \in \boldsymbol{R}^4$ in homogeneous coordinates as $\boldsymbol{m}_i = (m_{i,x}, m_{i,y}, m_{i,z}, 1)^T \in \mathbb{R}^4$ with $i \in [1, N]$ and N the number of model points. This step is performed only once.

3 Catheter Segmentation

In the second step of our method, we segment the catheter in the fluoroscopic images. To this end, we first crop the image around the region of interest which is a 400×400 pixels region around the projected center of the catheter model. In the first frame, the position is know from the initialization step, in all subsequent frames, the tracking result from the previous frame is used. The next step is catheter segmentation, which will be explained shortly. After segmentation, the resulting image is thinned [18]. To obtain a smooth image for registration, the distance transform for the skeletonized image is calculated [19]. The image processing steps are summarized in Fig. 1.

The catheter segmentation method has to fulfill two requirements. First, it has to be reliable. Second, it has to be fast. Speed is necessary to ensure that the catheter can be tracked in real-time at the frame rate required by the physician. In our case, a combination of Haar-like features and a cascade of boosted classifiers can meet both demands. Haar-like features [20] calculate various patterns of intensity differences. Some features detect edges, whereas others focus on line-like structures which are useful for detecting the catheter, as it is a thin object. Several feature prototypes are listed in Fig. 2(a). Actual features are obtained by shifting and scaling the prototypes within a predefined window. Thereby, contextual information around the center pixel is considered, which is important to differentiate between catheter and background structures. These features can be calculated efficiently through integral images.

Even for moderate window sizes, the resulting number of features is large and easily amounts to several hundreds of thousands. In order to achieve reliable

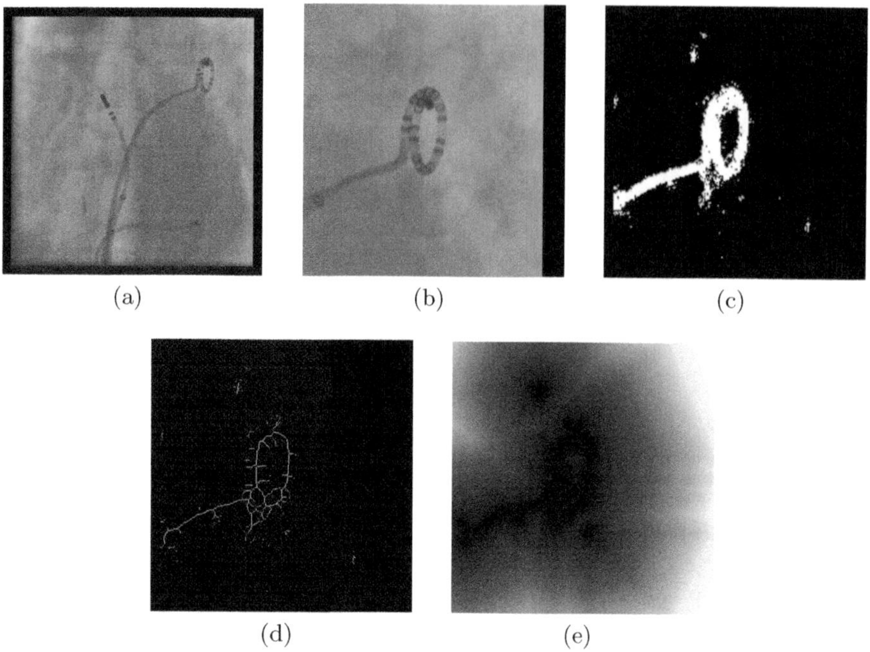

Fig. 1. (a) The original fluoroscopic input image. (b) Cropped image around the region-of-interest. (c) Segmentation using a boosted classifier cascade. (d) Skeletonized image. (e) Distance transformed image $\boldsymbol{I}_{\mathrm{DT}}$ to get a smooth image for registration.

and fast segmentation, the most suitable features for discriminating between catheter and background have to be chosen and integrated into a classifier in a suitable manner. This is carried out by the AdaBoost algorithm [21]. The idea is to combine several weak classifiers, which only have to be sligthly better than chance, to form a strong classifier. In the simplest case, a weak classifier amounts to a single feature and threshold. Weak classifiers are repeatedly evaluated on samples of a training set where the catheter has been annotated. The classifier minimizing the classification error is added to a linear combination of weak classifiers until the overall error is below the desired threshold. After each iteration, the importance of individual samples is re-weighted to put more emphasis on mis-classifications for the next evaluation.

Instead of single features and intensity thresholds, we use classification and regression trees (CARTs) [22] as weak classifiers. A CART is a small tree of fixed size. At each node, a threshold is associated with a feature partitioning the feature space. An example of a CART is shown in Fig. 2(b). Through this decomposition, flexibility is increased and objects with complex feature distributions can be handled.

Weighted combinations of CARTs are organized into a cascade, which is illustrated in Fig. 2(c). At each stage, a sample is either rejected or passed on to the next stage. Only if the sample is accepted at the final stage, it is assumed to

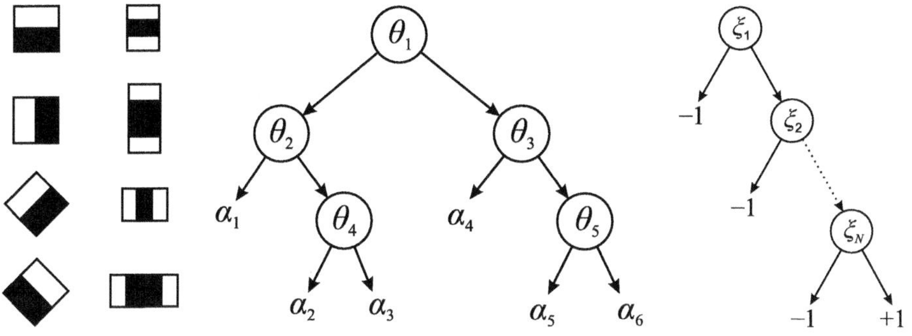

(a) Feature Types (b) Classification and Regression Tree (CART) (c) Cascade

Fig. 2. Features types and classifier structure for catheter segmentation: (a) several (lowpass) Haar filter examples used for feature extraction; (b) example of classification and regression tree (CART) with five feature nodes $\theta_1, \dots, \theta_5$ and six leaves $\alpha_1, \dots, \alpha_6$; (c) classifier cascade consisting of N stages with strong classifiers $\xi_1, \dots \xi_N$. Each strong classifier ξ_i consists of a linear combination of weak classifiers, here CARTs.

belong to the object. Thus, during training, the focus is on maintaining a high true positive rate while successively reducing the false positive rate, either by adding more weak classifiers to a stage or by adding an entirely new stage. For training, a gold-standard segmentation of the catheter was used.

4 Constrained Model-Based 2-D/3-D Registration

In the third step of our method, the actual motion compensation is performed by a constrained model-based 2-D/3-D registration. The catheter model is manually initialized in the first pair of frames of a biplane sequence and afterwards tracked throughout the remainder of one monoplane sequence. Tracking itself is performed by rigid 2-D/3-D registration. The constraint used for registration is that the search range is restricted to all directions parallel to the imaging plane. No search is performed perpendicular to the optical plane, i.e., along the optical axis. This is not a major issue, because shifts along the optical axis merely result in size changes of the motion-compensated fluoroscopic overlay. A motion analysis of the LA, performed by Ector et al. [23], revealed that the dominant motion is in anterior-posterior and superior-inferior direction. They found that the degree of rotation is much less, and they contributed it to the deformation of the left atrium. The mismatch in depth between the 3-D overlay and the live fluoroscopic images mainly results in small changes of the LA size which we found negligible for augmented fluoroscopy applications in clinical practice. Therefore, we focused on the remaining dominant motion directions in superior-inferior and lateral directions. To carry out this constrained 2-D/3-D registration, the viewing direction $\boldsymbol{n} \in \mathbb{R}^3$ with $||\boldsymbol{n}||_2 = 1$ is obtained from the projection matrix

$\boldsymbol{P} \in \mathbb{R}^{3\times 4}$. The viewing direction is perpendicular to all vectors that are parallel to the imaging plane. To calculate two spanning vectors of such a plane, an arbitrary vector $\boldsymbol{w} \in \boldsymbol{R}^3$ with $||\boldsymbol{w}||_2 = 1$ and $\boldsymbol{n}^T\boldsymbol{w} \neq 0$ is chosen. The spanning vectors $\boldsymbol{u}, \boldsymbol{v} \in \mathbb{R}^3$ of the search plane are then computed by

$$\boldsymbol{u} = \boldsymbol{n} \times \boldsymbol{w} \tag{6}$$

$$\boldsymbol{v} = \boldsymbol{n} \times \boldsymbol{u} \tag{7}$$

with $||\boldsymbol{u}||_2 = 1$ and $||\boldsymbol{v}||_2 = 1$. Depending on the choice of $\boldsymbol{w}$, the vectors $\boldsymbol{u}$ and $\boldsymbol{v}$ are different, but since these vectors span the same plane, any point on that plane can be represented by a linear combination of these two vectors. Moving a point $\boldsymbol{q} \in \mathbb{R}^3$ parallel to the imaging plane is achieved by

$$\boldsymbol{q}^\star = \boldsymbol{q} + \lambda\boldsymbol{u} + \mu\boldsymbol{v} \tag{8}$$

with the translated point $\boldsymbol{q}^\star \in \boldsymbol{R}^3$ and the amount of translation defined by $\lambda, \mu \in \mathbb{R}$.

We compute a transformation matrix $\boldsymbol{T}(\lambda, \mu) \in \boldsymbol{R}^{4\times 4}$ as

$$\boldsymbol{T}(\lambda, \mu) = \begin{pmatrix} 1 & 0 & 0 & \lambda u_x + \mu v_x \\ 0 & 1 & 0 & \lambda u_y + \mu v_y \\ 0 & 0 & 1 & \lambda u_z + \mu v_z \\ 0 & 0 & 0 & 1 \end{pmatrix} \tag{9}$$

with $\boldsymbol{u} = (u_x, u_y, u_z)^T$ and $\boldsymbol{v} = (v_x, v_y, v_z)^T$. The objective function for the constrained registration is then defined by using the values of the distance transformed image $\boldsymbol{I}_{\mathrm{DT}}$ as cost function by

$$\hat{\lambda}, \hat{\mu} = \arg\min_{\lambda,\mu} \sum_i \boldsymbol{I}_{\mathrm{DT}}\left(\boldsymbol{P} \cdot \boldsymbol{T}(\lambda, \mu) \cdot \boldsymbol{m}_i\right). \tag{10}$$

Rotation is not considered, as we are primarily interested in the compensation of breathing motion which occurs in axial direction. The projection matrix considered for projecting the model into the imaging plane is not required to be one of the projection matrices used for model generation, i.e., the C-arm can be moved in between model generation and tracking. Given the parameters $\hat{\lambda}, \hat{\mu}$, found by a nearest-neighbor search, that minimize Eq. (10), the catheter model can be updated to $\boldsymbol{m}_i^\star \in \boldsymbol{R}^4$ by

$$\forall i : \boldsymbol{m}_i^\star = \boldsymbol{T}(\lambda, \mu) \cdot \boldsymbol{m}_i. \tag{11}$$

The same transformation $\boldsymbol{T}(\hat{\lambda}, \hat{\mu})$ is then also applied to the 3-D volumetric data set that is used for the image overlay. This way, we can achieve a 3-D motion compensation for mono-plane fluoroscopic images.

5 Evaluation and Results

Evaluation was performed using a leave-one-out validation approach. The tracking accuracy was measured in comparison to a gold-standard segmentation.

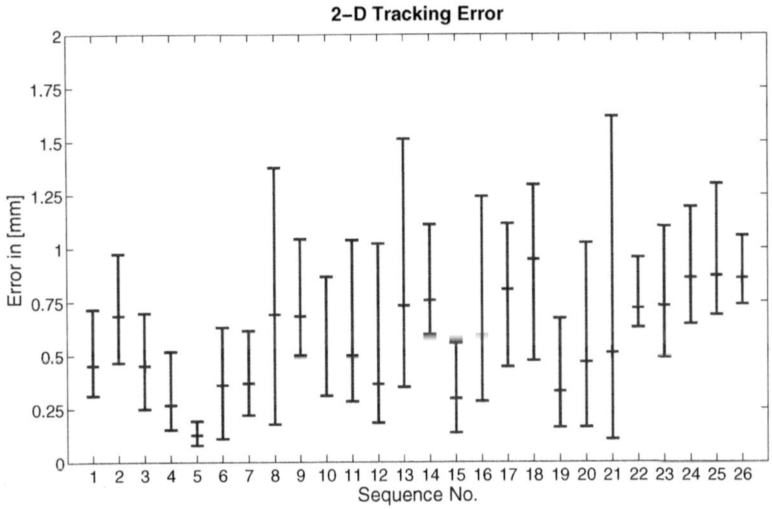

Fig. 3. Two-dimensional tracking error for all 26 sequences. For each sequence, the average error, minimum error, and maximum error is given. An overall mean error of 0.58 mm, an overall minimum error of 0.08 mm, and an overall maximum error of 1.62 mm was achieved.

The sequence considered for testing was not included in the respective training data set. For evaluation, 13 clinical biplane sequences were available. Our data was taken from six different patients at one clinical site. They were recorded on an AXIOM Artis dBC biplane C-arm system (Siemens AG, Healthcare, Forchheim, Germany). For each sequence, a 3-D model was generated as described in Sec. 2. Afterwards, our method was evaluated by considering each imaging plane of the biplane sequences independently. This way, we obtained 26 sequences with a total frame number of 938 frames to evaluate catheter tracking. A 2-D tracking error was obtained by calculating the average 2-D distance of the projected catheter model to the gold-standard segmentation used for training. The average error, minimum error, and maximum error for each sequence are illustrated in Fig. 3. Our method yielded an overall mean error of 0.58 mm, an overall minimum error of 0.08 mm, and an overall maximum error of 1.62 mm.

Since the motion compensation is performed in 3-D, a 3-D error can estimated as well. To this end, the tip of circumferential mapping catheter was manually localized in 3-D using triangulation from two views. The available 3-D trajectories of the catheter tip were taken as a gold-standard for the observed 3-D motion.

In one sequence, the 3-D error turned out rather high, because the catheter moved significantly perpendicular to the optical plane, see Fig. 4. However, in cases where the circumferential mapping catheter was firmly placed at a pulmonary vein no such movement occurred, and we were able move the overlay well in sync with the 3-D motion. The method in [16] is still superior regarding

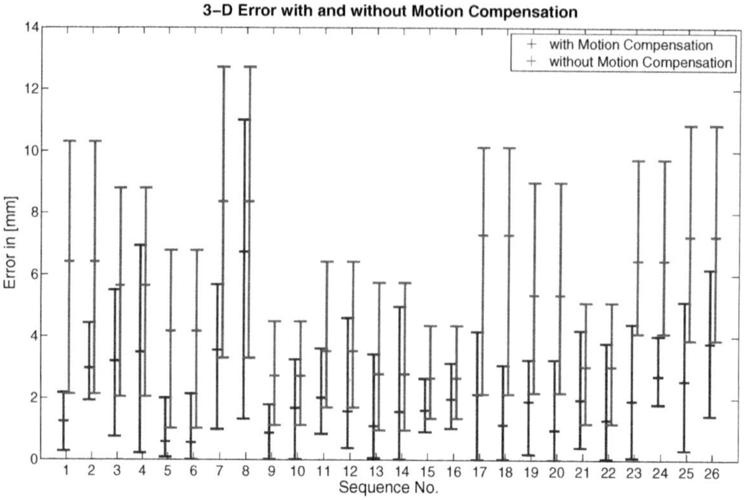

Fig. 4. Three-dimensional tracking error for all 26 sequences in comparison to the observed 3-D motion. For each sequence, the average, minimum, and maximum for the tracking error as well as the observed motion is given. On average, we observed an overall mean error of 2.12 mm, an overall minimum error of 0.01 mm, and an overall maximum error of 11.01 mm was achieved.

the 3-D error, but its better accuracy comes at the cost of simultaneous biplane fluorosopy, i.e., increased X-ray dose.

6 Discussion and Conclusions

The 2-D tracking error of our proposed method is in the same range as 2-D reference method [15]. But instead of performing only a 2-D/2-D registration, we now rely on a constrained 2-D/3-D registration involving a 3-D catheter model. The advantage of a 3-D catheter model is that re-positioning of the C-arm is possible whereas a 2-D catheter representation needs to be re-initialized if view directions change. Nevertheless, a pure 2-D approach is the method of choice if only a monoplane fluoroscopic system is available. In addition, our new approach is learning-based whereas the approach in [15] is filter-based. Therefore, our new method requires a training phase for the segmentation of the catheter. Note, however, that by using a learning-based method we might be able to improve the tracking results. At least, this is what we observed for the biplane approach [14]. Here, the filter-based approach [16] yielded a 2-D tracking error of 1.0 mm and a 3-D tracking error of 0.8 mm. Using a learning-based method, the errors were reduced to 0.8 mm in 2-D and to 0.7 mm in 3-D [14].

The dedicated biplane method [14] yields a smaller 3-D error than our new method, but it requires simultaneously biplane fluoroscopy. A comparison of all three methods (current approach, [14], [15]) is given in Tab. 1. In our current

Table 1. Comparison between available methods for respiratory and cardiac motion compensation during atrial fibrillation catheter ablation procedures. Our method uses a learning-based approach to segment a commonly used circumferential mapping catheter and then performs a mono-plane 2-D/3-D registration of a 3-D model to the segmentation. The method in [14] a bi-plane 2-D/3-D registration. The method in [15] uses a filter-based method to segment the same catheter and uses only a 2-D model which is registered to mono-plane sequences.

Method Comparison			
	Our	**[14]**	**[15]**
Catheter Model	3-D	3-D	2-D
Compensation in	3-D	3-D	2-D
mono-/biplane fluoro	+/+	-/+	+/-
Mean 2-D Error:	0.58 mm	0.8 mm	0.59 mm
Mean 3-D Error:	2.12 mm	0.7 mm	—

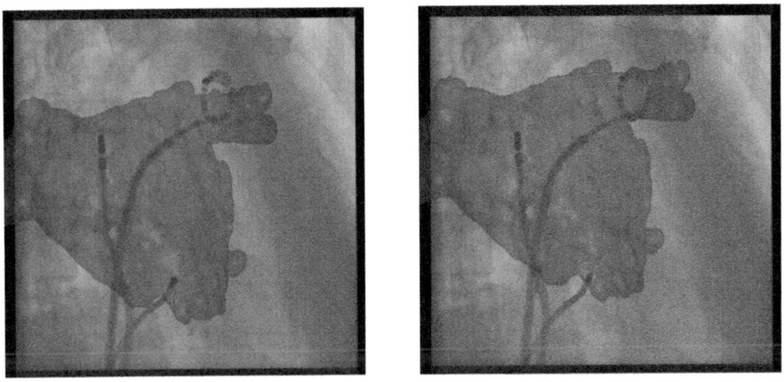

(a) (b)

Fig. 5. A comparison showing the difference if motion compensation is considered or not. (a) One frame of sequence 17 without motion compensation. (b) Shows the same frame of sequence 17 as in (a) but this time with motion compensation.

technique, we provide only a limited 3-D motion compensation but do not require simultaneously biplane fluoroscopy as in [14]. The limitation of our method is mainly related to the fact that motion along the viewing direction cannot be taken into account as depth information is hard to determine from mono-plane projection images. To achieve a depth correction, a perfect segmentation of the catheter would be required and, in addition, we would also need to know the exact dimensions of the catheter in 3-D, i.e., its diameter and its thickness. Any noise in the 2-D segmentation or at the 3-D model would decrease the accuracy of the depth estimate. To avoid this problem we have chosen to use only search directions parallel to the imaging plane. As a price to pay, we accept that the 3-D error will not be as good as in [15]. As in the previously presented methods, our new approach does not require a perfect segmentation of the circumferential mapping catheter, because the registration method can compensate for segmentation errors.

For comparison, electro-anatomic mapping systems provide a mean tracking error of 0.7 mm [24] which is comparable to our mean tracking error of 0.58 mm. In addition, our reference catheter, the circumferential mapping catheter, is directly at the site of ablation. Hence, it enables motion compensation for respiratory and cardiac motion without the need to separate these two motion patterns or the requirement to synchronize with ECG. Since we do not need to record the ECG signal, a stand-alone version of an augmented-reality, motion-compensated fluoroscopy system is possible.

A comparison between a frame with and without motion compensation is presented in Fig. 5. In a clinical setup, a physician working on a biplane system is likely to use his imaging planes in an alternating way. For such a clinical use case, our newly proposed method provides a significant advantage over the previously introduced methods [13,15] in terms of accuracy and practicality.

Acknowledgements

This work has been supported by the German Federal Ministry of Education and Research in the context of the initiative Spitzencluster Medical Valley - Europäische Metropolregion Nürnberg. Additional funding was provided by Siemens Healthcare.

References

1. Gage, B., Waterman, A., Shannon, W., Boechler, M., Rich, M., Radford, M.: Validation of Clinical Classification Schemes for Predicting Stroke. JAMA 285(22), 2864–2870 (2001)
2. Haissaguerre, M., Gencel, L., Fischer, B., Le Metayer, P., Poquet, F., Marcus, F., Clementy, J.: Successful Catheter Ablation of Atrial Fibrillation. J. Cardiovasc Electrophysiol. 5, 1045–1052 (1994)
3. Calkins, H., Brugada, J., Packer, D., Cappato, R., Chen, S., Crijns, H., Damiano, R., Davies, D., Haines, D., Haissaguerre, M., Iesaka, Y., Jackman, W., Jais, P., Kottkamp, H., Kuck, K., Lindsay, B., Marchlinski, F., McCarthy, P., Mont, J., Moradi, F., Nademanee, K., Natale, A., Pappone, C., Prystowsky, E., Raviele, A., Ruskin, J., Shemin, R.: HRS/EHRA/ECAS Expert Consensus Statement on Catheter and Surgical Ablation of Atrial Fibrillation: Recommendations for Personnel, Policy, Procedures and Follow-Up. Europace 9(6), 335–379 (2007)
4. Prümmer, M., Wigström, L., Hornegger, J., Boese, J., Lauritsch, G., Strobel, N., Fahrig, R.: Cardiac C-arm CT: Efficient Motion Correction for 4D-FBP. In: IEEE Nuclear Science Symposium Conference Record (2006)
5. Wittkampf, F., Wever, E., Derksen, R., Wilde, A., Ramanna, H., Hauer, R., Robles de Medina, E.: LocaLisa - New Technique for Real-Time 3-Dimensional Localization of Regular Intracardiac Electrodes. Circulation 99(13), 1312–1317 (1999)
6. Kistler, P., Rajappan, K., Jahngir, M., Earley, M., Harris, S., Abrams, D., Gupta, D., Liew, R., Ellis, S., Sporton, S., Schilling, R.: The Impact of CT Image Integration into an Electroanatomic Mapping System on Clinical Outcomes of Catheter

Ablation of Atrial Fibrillation. Journal of Cardiovascular Electrophysiology 17(10), 1093–1101 (2006)

7. Kistler, P.M., Earley, M.J., Harris, S., Abrams, D., Ellis, S., Sporton, S.C., Schilling, R.J.: Validation of Three-Dimensional Cardiac Image Integration: Use of Integrated CT Image into Electroanatomic Mapping System to Perform Catheter Ablation of Atrial Fibrillation. Journal of Cardiovascular Electrophysiology 17(4), 341–348 (2006)
8. Kistler, P.M., Rajappan, K., Harris, S., Earley, M.J., Richmond, L., Sporton, S.C., Schilling, R.J.: The impact of image integration on catheter ablation of atrial fibrillation using electroanatomic mapping: a prospective randomized study. European Heart Journal 29(24), 3029–3036 (2008)
9. Daccarett, M., Segerson, N., Günther, J., Nölker, G., Gutleben, K., Brachmann, J., Marrouche, N.: Blinded correlation study of three-dimensional electro-anatomical image integration and phased array intra-cardiac echocardiography for left atrial mapping. Europace 9, 923–926 (2007)
10. Ector, J., De Buck, S., Huybrechts, W., Nuyens, D., Dymarkowski, S., Bogaert, J., Maes, F., Heidbüchel, H.: Biplane three-dimensional augmented fluoroscopy as single navigation tool for ablation of atrial fibrillation: Accuracy and clinical value. Heart Rhythm 5(7), 957–964 (2008)
11. Sra, J., Narayan, G., Krum, D., Malloy, A., Cooley, R., Bhatia, A., Dhala, A., Blanck, Z., Nangia, V., Akhtar, M.: Computed Tomography-Fluoroscopy Image Integration-Guided Catheter Ablation of Atrial Fibrillation. J. Cardiovasc Electrophysiol. 18(4), 409–414 (2007)
12. De Buck, S., Maes, F., Ector, J., Bogaert, J., Dymarkowski, S., Heidbüchel, H., Suetens, P.: An Augmented Reality System for Patient-Specific Guidance of Cardiac Catheter Ablation Procedures. IEEE Transactions on Medical Imaging 24(11), 1512–1524 (2005)
13. Brost, A., Liao, R., Hornegger, J., Strobel, N.: 3-D respiratory motion compensation during EP procedures by image-based 3-D lasso catheter model generation and tracking. In: Yang, G.-Z., Hawkes, D., Rueckert, D., Noble, A., Taylor, C. (eds.) MICCAI 2009. LNCS, vol. 5761, pp. 394–401. Springer, Heidelberg (2009)
14. Brost, A., Wimmer, A., Liao, R., Hornegger, J., Strobel, N.: Catheter tracking: Filter-based vs. Learning-based. In: Goesele, M., Roth, S., Kuijper, A., Schiele, B., Schindler, K. (eds.) Pattern Recognition. LNCS, vol. 6376, pp. 293–302. Springer, Heidelberg (2010)
15. Brost, A., Liao, R., Hornegger, J., Strobel, N.: Model-based registration for motion compensation during EP ablation procedures. In: Fischer, B., Dawant, B.M., Lorenz, C. (eds.) WBIR 2010. LNCS, vol. 6204, pp. 234–245. Springer, Heidelberg (2010)
16. Brost, A., Liao, R., Strobel, N., Hornegger, J.: Respiratory motion compensation by model-based catheter tracking during EP procedures. Medical Image Analysis 14(5), 695–706 (2010); Special Issue on the 12th International Conference on Medical Image Computing and Computer-Assisted Intervention (MICCAI) 2009
17. Quan, L.: Conic Reconstruction and Correspondence From Two Views. IEEE Trans. Pattern Anal. Mach. Intell. 18(2), 151–160 (1996)
18. Cychosz, J.: Efficient Binary Image Thinning using Neighborhood Maps. Graphics Gems IV, 465–473 (1994)
19. Breu, H., Gil, J., Kirkpatrick, D., Werman, M.: Linear time Euclidean distance transform algorithms. IEEE Trans. Pattern Anal. Mach. Intell. 17, 529–533 (1995)
20. Viola, P., Jones, M.: Robust real-time face detection. Int. J. Comput. Vision 57(2), 137–154 (2004)

21. Freund, Y., Schapire, R.: A decision-theoretic generalization of on-line learning and an application to boosting. JCSS 55(1), 119–139 (1997)
22. Breiman, L., Friedman, J., Olshen, R., Stone, C.: Classification and Regression Trees. Chapman & Hall, New York (1984)
23. Ector, J., De Buck, S., Loeckx, D., Coudyzer, W., Maes, F., Dymarkowski, S., Bogaert, J., Heidbüchel, H.: Changes in left atrial anatomy due to respiration: Impact on three-dimensional image integration during atrial fibrillation ablation. J. Cardiovasc Electrophysiol. 19(8), 828–834 (2008)
24. Gepstein, L., Hayam, G., Ben-Haim, S.: A Novel Method for Nonfluoroscopic Catheter-Based Electroanatomical Mapping of the Heart: In Vitro and In Vivo Accuracy Results. Circulation 95, 1611–1622 (1997)

Image-Based Automatic Ablation Point Tagging System with Motion Correction for Cardiac Ablation Procedures

YingLiang Ma[1], Gang Gao[1], Geert Gijsbers[2], C. Aldo Rinaldi[3], Jaswinder Gill[3], Reza Razavi[1], and Kawal S. Rhode[1]

[1] Division of Imaging Sciences and Biomedical Engineering, King's College London, SE1 7EH, UK
[2] Philips Healthcare, Best, The Netherlands
[3] Department of Cardiology, Guy's & St. Thomas' Hospitals NHS Foundation Trust, London, SE1 7EH, UK
y.ma@kcl.ac.uk

Abstract. X-ray fluoroscopically guided cardiac ablation procedures are commonly carried out for the treatment of cardiac arrhythmias, such as atrial fibrillation (AF). X-ray images have poor soft tissue contrast and, for this reason, overlay of a 3D roadmap derived from pre-procedural volumetric image data can be used to add anatomical information. It is a requirement to determine and record the 3D positions of the ablation catheter tip in the 3D road map during AF ablation. This feature can be used as a guidance and post-procedure analysis tool. The 3D positions of the catheter tip can be calculated from biplane X-ray images and mapped to the 3D roadmap. However, the registration between the 3D roadmap and the 2D X-ray data can be compromised by patient respiratory and cardiac motions. As the coronary sinus (CS) catheter is not routinely altered during the procedure, tracking the CS catheter in real-time can be used as means of motion correction to improve the accuracy of registration between live X-ray images and a 3D roadmap. To achieve a fast and automatic ablation point tagging system from biplane images, we developed a novel tracking method for real-time simultaneous detection of the ablation catheter and the CS catheter from fluoroscopic X-ray images. We tested our tracking method on 1083 fluoroscopy frames from 16 patients and achieved a success rate of 97.5% and an average 2D tracking error of 0.5 mm ± 0.3 mm. In order to achieve tagging using a mono-plane X-ray image system, we proposed a novel motion gating method to select a pair of images from two short image sequences acquired from two different views. Both respiratory and cardiac motion phases are matched by selecting the pair of images with the minimum reconstruction error of the CS catheter electrodes. Finally, the 3D position of the ablation catheter tip was calculated using the epipolar constraint from the multiview images. We validated our automatic ablation point tagging strategy by computing the reconstruction error of the ablation catheter tip and achieved an error of 1.1 mm ± 0.5 mm.

1 Introduction

Atrial fibrillation (AF) is one of the most common cardiac arrhythmias, affecting 2.2 million patients in the U.S. alone. It can be treated using catheter-based radiofrequency ablation (RFA) therapy. During this procedure, an ablation catheter is

R.H. Taylor and G.-Z. Yang (Eds.): IPCAI 2011, LNCS 6689, pp. 145–155, 2011.

inserted into a heart chamber (usually the left atrium for AF) and the RF energy is delivered via the catheter tip to create myocardial lesions, thereby disrupting the local electrical activity. AF ablation procedures are traditionally carried out under X-ray fluoroscopic guidance. However, X-ray images have poor soft tissue contrast and it is difficult to interpret the anatomical context directly from these images. To overcome the lack of soft tissue contrast, a three-dimensional (3D) roadmap can be generated from 3D high-resolution computed tomography (CT)/ magnetic resonance images (MRI), registered and overlaid in real-time with X-ray fluoroscopy images [1] (see figure 1a). Modern cardiac interventional X-ray systems [2] can also performance CT-like imaging by fast rotation of the C-arm with contrast agent injection, a process known as C-arm CT [3] or rotational X-ray angiography (RXA) [4]. Roadmaps can be generated from C-arm CT/RXA data and also overlaid on to X-ray fluoroscopy for interventional guidance [5]. 3D image-derived anatomical overlay is now a widely accepted method for guiding ablation procedures with this technology available from all major imaging manufacturers [6]. It is a very useful function to determine and record the 3D positions of the ablation catheter tip in the 3D road map (see figure 1a) during the AF ablation procedure. This feature can be used for ablation guidance and post-procedure analysis. There are a few commercial ablation catheter tip tracking and ablation point tagging systems currently available to perform this task such as CARTO (Biosense Webster Inc., CA, USA) and Ensite NavX (St Jude Medical, MN, USA). The errors for the CARTO and Ensite NavX systems have previously been investigated using phantoms or controlled animal experiments. The reported accuracy ranges from 1.9 to 6.6 mm [7]. However, both these systems require special hardware and catheters. The additional costs are substantial compared with using X-ray fluoroscopic guidance coupled to an overlaid 3D roadmap. In order to achieve recording (tagging) of the 3D position of the ablation points using X-ray fluoroscopic guidance, two technical challenges have to be solved. The first is robust and fast image-based ablation catheter tip tracking. A technique of tracking electrophysiology catheters in X-ray images was proposed by Franken et al. [8]. The success rate of tracking the catheter tip was up to 80% in low does X-ray fluoroscopic images and the computational cost was relatively high. We present a novel technique to track the ablation catheter tip from X-ray images in real-time. This technique uses a fast blob detection method to detect all possible electrode-like objects in the X-ray image and then search for the ablation catheter. The main novelty of our technique is that we combine a catheter tip shape model with a catheter geometry model that includes features such as the number of electrodes, distance constraints and angle constraints. This prior knowledge of the ablation catheter could allow the rapid and robust distinction of the ablation catheter from other catheters and instruments in the X-ray image. Our tracking method uses the whole image as a region of interest so that we are able to track the ablation catheter even in the presence of large sudden motion. Furthermore, the proposed method does not require any user interaction.

The second challenge is the development of robust, fast image-based motion correction and gating methods. Currently, in X-ray fluoroscopic overlay guidance the 3D roadmap remains static and does not move with the patient's respiratory and cardiac motions. In some cases, respiratory motion can cause a two-dimensional (2D) registration error of over 14 mm [9], which is a significant compromise in the accuracy of guidance. In order to achieve clinical acceptable accuracy, a motion correction method should be used. Image-based methods are preferred as we aim to use the X-ray fluoroscopic images. A number of groups have addressed the issue of respiratory and/or cardiac motion correction or gating in the literature. Shechter et al. [10] constructed a model of cardiac and respiratory motion of the coronary arteries from biplane contrast-enhanced X-ray image sequences. The model was applied by tracking the motion of the diaphragm in subsequent (non-enhanced) X-ray images. However, forming the model from X-ray images under contrast injection means that it will be constructed from a limited amount of data. Furthermore, the diaphragm is not always in the X-ray field of view, particularly for obese patients. Sundar et al. [11] proposed an automatic image-based cardiac and respiratory motion gating method by calculating the cumulated phase shift in the spectral domain from X-ray fluoroscopic image sequences. This method is based on detection of the energy change in the images. The energy change could be caused by the motion of catheters or contrast agent injection, for example. As the method uses overall motion of moving objects, the cardiac and respiratory cycle motions detected by this method could be erroneous when the clinician manipulates the catheters or injects contrast agent. Brost et al. [12] developed an image-based respiratory motion correction method for EP procedures by tracking a lasso catheter from X-ray fluoroscopic images. Tracking the lasso catheter makes this method robust against movement of other catheters. However, it also has some limitations. Firstly, the lasso catheter does not always remain stationary inside the heart. Secondly, the tracking method required manual initialization. In our previous paper [13], we developed a real-time method to track the coronary sinus (CS) catheter from X-ray images. In this study, we use CS catheter not only as the real-time motion correction tool but also as the novel tool for motion gating from a mono-plane X-ray system. The biplane system is the ideal platform for tagging 3D position of the ablation catheter tip. However, the majority of interventional cardiology X-ray systems are single plane systems. Therefore, a novel motion gating method using the CS catheter tracking was developed to select a pair of X-ray images from two short X-ray fluoroscopic image sequences by matching the phases of both cardiac and respiratory cycle motions. Two short X-ray image sequences are acquired from two different angles using the mono-plane X-ray system. In this paper, we reference the selected pair of X-ray images as the biplane X-ray images. Finally, we are able to compute the 3D position of the ablation catheter tip from biplane X-ray images using the epipolar constraint [14] and map it on the surface of the 3D roadmap.

2 Method

A typical catheter setup for an AF ablation procedure contains one ablation catheter, one lasso catheter and one CS catheter. Tracking the ablation catheter in real-time is much more difficult than CS catheter tracking because the ablation catheter can stay very close to the lasso catheter and overlap with it. Therefore, we use a shape model of the catheter tip and a geometry model to distinguish the ablation catheter from other catheters (particularly the lasso catheter).

2.1 Ablation Catheter Tracking

Similar to the first step of the CS catheter tracking method in [13], we use a blob detector based on the determinant of the Hessian matrix [15], which is defined as

$$\det H(L(x,y;t)) = t^2 (L_{xx} L_{yy} - L_{xy}^2) \tag{1}$$

where $L(x,y;t) = I(x,y) * g(x,y;t)$ is the scale-space representation of the image $I(x,y)$ with the scale fact t and $g(x,y;t)$ is the Gaussian filter. $L_{xx} = I(x,y) * g_{xx}$ and similar definitions apply for L_{yy} and L_{xy}. g_{xx}, g_{yy} and g_{xy} are Gaussian derivatives and also known as Laplacian of Gaussians (LoG). In practice, we just pre-compute the masks of these Gaussian derivatives, convolve with the input image and calculate the determinant of the Hessian matrix. Blobs are detected as regional maxima of the determinant of the Hessian matrix and we also define the strength of the blob as the normalized value of the determinant of the Hessian matrix. In addition, we compute the first eigen vector of the Hessian matrix to find out the orientation of large blobs. They are likely to be the catheter tip electrodes. Finally, we need to decide the scale factors t for detecting catheter electrodes. Four fixed scale factors are used to detect electrodes on CS and ablation catheters as we design a method that tracks not only the ablation catheter but also the CS catheter at the same time. As shown in figure 1b, the ablation catheter tip electrode is larger than CS catheter tip electrode and other electrodes on the ablation catheter are also bigger. Therefore, there are two fixed scale factors for the ablation catheter and two other fixed scale factors for the CS catheter. To calculate the scale factor t, we use $t = (s/3)^2$ where s is the size of blob. This equation is motivated by the "3σ" ($t = \sigma^2$) rule that 99% of energy of the Gaussian is within three standard deviations. The value of the blob size s was set to 8 or 4 pixels for the CS catheter tip electrode and the smaller electrodes and was set to 16 or 6 pixels for ablation catheter tip electrode and the smaller electrodes, respectively. This was estimated for a 512 × 512 X-ray image with a pixel to mm ratio, R_{xray}, at 0.25. Figure 1c demonstrates the result of blob detection in a low-dose X-ray image.

To estimate the ratio R_{xray} in X-ray images, the pixel to mm ratio $R_{\det}$ from X-ray detector is used. Although $R_{\det}$ gives the ratio from pixel to mm, it is only correct when the magnification factor M of X-ray system is 1.0. To calculate the magnification factor M, the following assumptions were used: (1) the patient heart was aligned to the iso-center of X-ray system; and (2) the X-ray system was calibrated. Assumption (1) is assured by the clinical protocol and (2) is assured by the routine maintenance of the system. The magnification factor M is computed using $M = D_{\det}/D_{pat}$, where $D_{\det}$ is the distance from X-ray source to the detector and D_{pat} is the distance from X-ray source to the patient. Finally, $R_{xray} = R_{\det}/M$.

The next step uses a catheter tip shape model and a catheter geometry model to decide which combination of blobs represents the ablation catheter. The ablation catheter has a large and solid catheter tip electrode which casts a dark, solid and thin ellipse-like blob in the X-ray images (see figure 1b). Therefore, we build a simple

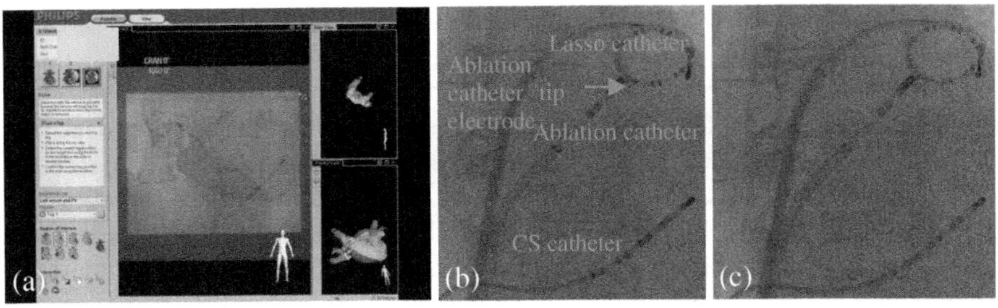

Fig. 1. a) Example of an anatomical overlay with ablation point tagging. b) Original low-dose X-ray image. c) The result from the blob detection method. Red crosses are the positions of electrode-like blobs.

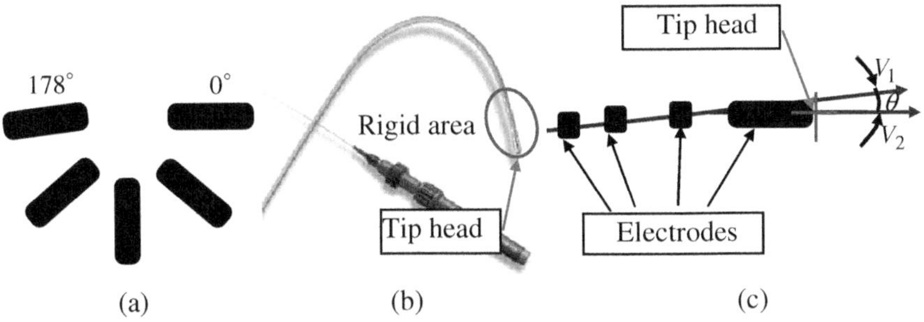

Fig. 2. a) Ablation catheter tip templates in different orientations. b) The ablation catheter. The rigid area is within red circle. c) The definition of the turning angle.

black template for it based on the estimated size and pre-compute it in different orientations. We only rotate the template from 0 degrees to 178 degrees with a step of 2 degrees as the template is symmetric (see figure 2a). After the blob detection method gives the positions of the candidate catheter tip blobs and the first eigen vector of the Hessian matrix, the template in the closest orientation with the first eigen vector is selected. Then this selected template is translated along the first and second eigen vectors to find the optimal position by using a normalized cross correlation (NCC) algorithm. As the template is symmetric and the catheter tip blob in the X-ray image is likely symmetric along tip head and tip foot direction, both the first eigen vector and template matching can not reliably locate the tip head (see figure 2b and 2c) where the ablation of heart muscle tissue takes place. It can be easily flipped 180 degrees to locate the tip foot as the tip head.

Therefore, we further use a search algorithm to decide which combination of blobs represents the ablation catheter. The search algorithm used for CS catheter tracking [13] fails for ablation catheter tracking as the lasso catheter often stays close and overlaps with the ablation catheter. However, by studying the physical properties of the ablation catheter, we find out that the region of the catheter tip and its other three electrodes is very rigid (see figure 2b) and cannot make a turning angle of more than 30 degrees. The turning angle is defined as θ in figure 2c. This finding was confirmed by studying our 1083 X-ray fluoroscopic images acquired during 16 cases of

AF ablation procedures. The search algorithm starts with selecting the 50 highest strength blobs from the blob detection method and they are sorted by strength from strongest to weakest. The number 50 was empirically determined and relates to the maximum number of likely blob-like structures present in typical X-ray data. Those blobs are used as candidates for catheter electrodes. Then the search algorithm of CS catheter tracking is used to indentify which combination of blobs represents a CS catheter. Blobs from CS catheter are removed from the list of 50 highest strength blobs. The first 5 strongest blobs are selected as the candidates for the ablation catheter tip and then the template matching is applied to all 5 blobs. Template matching uses NCC and produces a matching score S_{NCC}, which is normalized to between 0 and 1. Finally, from the optimal position of tip electrode center provided by template matching, we start to search for the other three electrodes along the direction and the opposite direction of the first eigen vector. The reason for searching two directions is the symmetry of ablation catheter tip. Two constraints are applied to the searching. One is the turning angle θ. 30 degrees is the maximum value of θ. The second constraint is the maximum gap between two electrodes. There are some variations of maximum gap between two electrodes of the ablation catheters from several manufacturers. We just choose the maximum one (5 mm) among them and the cut-off threshold is the twice that value. It is 10 mm or 40 pixels (based on the pixel to mm ratio at 0.25). Finally, a cost function is designed to estimate the likelihood of ablation catheter like objects. The ablation catheter like objects should have a large blob as the catheter tip and several smaller blobs after it. The cost function is defined as follows

$$ABCathCost = (1 - Blob_{tip}) + S_{NCC} + \left\|1 - \cos\theta\right\| + \frac{4 - NumOfBlobs}{4} \quad (2)$$

where $Blob_{tip}$ is the strength of catheter tip like blob which is computed as the normalized determination of the Hessian matrix and its range is from 0 to 1. S_{NCC} is the score of normalized cross correlation. θ is the turning angle. $\cos\theta$ can be computed efficiently using $\cos\theta_i = \vec{V_1} \bullet \vec{V_2} / \left(\left\|\vec{V_1}\right\| \cdot \left\|\vec{V_2}\right\|\right)$, where $\bullet$ is the dot product and $\|\ \|$ is the vector length. $\vec{V_1}$ is the direction vector of last two electrodes and $\vec{V_2}$ is the orientation vector of catheter tip which is determined by the first eigen vector of Hessian matrix. Both definitions are illustrated in figure 2c. The flow chart of overall ablation catheter tracking algorithm is shown in figure 3.

2.2 Motion Gating Using CS Catheter

Biplane images from a biplane X-ray system are an ideal image source for tagging the 3D positions of the ablation points as biplane images are synchronized in both respiratory and cardiac cycle motion phases. However, the majority of interventional cardiology X-ray systems are mono-plane system. Therefore, we designed a novel motion gating method to find a pair of images in similar respiratory and cardiac cycle motion phases from two short X-ray fluoroscopic image sequences. They are acquired from two different angle views using a mono-plane X-ray system when both the ablation catheter and CS catheter remain stationary. Typically, one is the posteroanterior (PA)

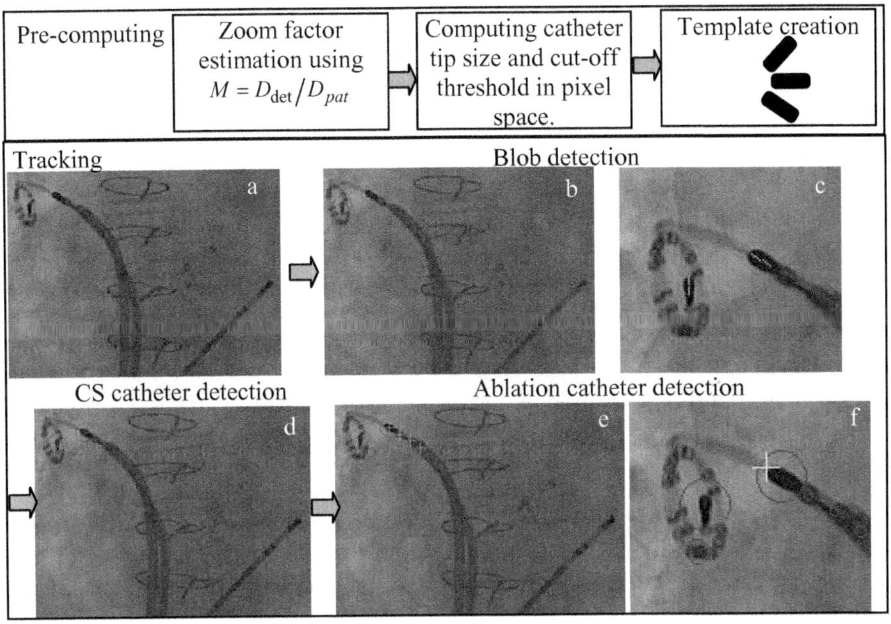

Fig. 3. The flow chart of overall ablation catheter tracking algorithm. a) The original X-ray image. b) Red crosses are the positions of blobs. The size of the red circles represents the strength of the blobs. c) The orientation vectors of large blobs (the first eigen vector of Hessian matrix). (d) The blue crosses are the positions of CS catheter electrodes. (e) Green crosses are the position of ablation catheter electrodes. (f) The yellow cross is the detected position of ablation catheter tip head.

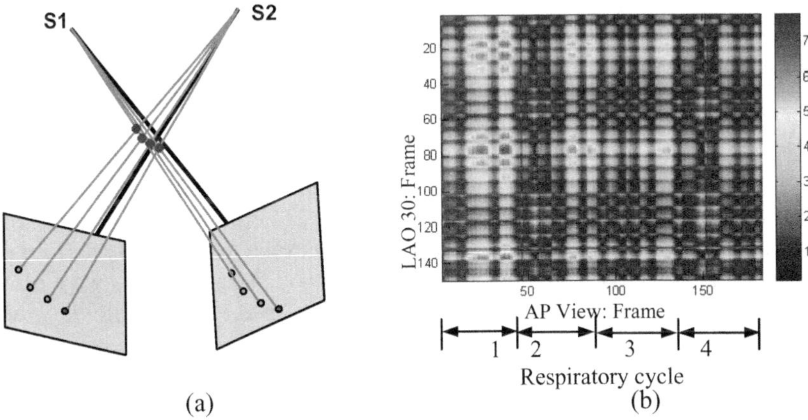

Fig. 4. a) 3D reconstruction using the epipolar constraint. b) The error matrix of reconstruction errors of the proximal electrode of CS catheter. The values in the color bar are in pixel units.

view and the other is the left/right anterior oblique (LAO/RAO) view. We reference this pair of images also as the biplane X-ray images. To search the pair of images, the CS catheter is tracked in every frame of the two sequences. For each possible pair of images from two views, the 3D position of the proximal electrode of the 10-electrode CS catheter is reconstructed using the epipolar constraint (figure 4a) and the 3D point is the mid-point of the shortest line segment connecting the two epipolar lines. The reason for choosing the proximal electrode of the CS catheter (the distal electrode is the catheter tip) is that the proximal electrode has lower tracking errors than the other electrodes. After computing the 3D position of the proximal electrode, the 3D point is projected back to the two image planes to obtain two 2D projected points. The 2D error is defined as the distance between the projected point and the original 2D position of the proximal electrode in one X-ray image view. The reconstruction error of the 3D point is defined as the maximum of the two 2D errors. An error matrix (figure 4b) is computed as the reconstruction errors among all possible pairs of X-ray images. Figure 4b used two long sequences to demonstrate our technique. In practice, two short sequences are only required. One needs only 2 to 5 frames (less than 1 second). The other one only requires the acquisition time of one breathing cycle. Finally, the motion gating is achieved by selecting a pair of images with a minimum reconstruction error. The 3D position of the ablation catheter tip head is computed from this pair of images and mapped onto the surface of the 3D roadmap and the 3D roadmap is constantly moved with the motion of the proximal electrode of CS catheter.

3 Results

We first tested the proposed ablation catheter tracking method on 1083 clinical X-ray images. There were a total of 57 different clinical fluoroscopy sequences which came from 16 AF ablation clinical cases. 49% of the clinical X-ray images that we tested were low dose and contained high frequency noise. Typically, the clinical X-ray images contained one CS catheter, one ablation catheter and one lasso catheter. Some X-ray fluoroscopy images contained sternal wire loops (figure 3a), which patients had from previous open-heart surgery.

3.1 Accuracy, Robustness and Efficiency Test of the Tracking Method

To test the accuracy of the ablation catheter tracking method, we asked two clinical experts to manually pick the centre position of the ablation catheter tip head on all 1083 images. Then we calculated the 2D distance between the manually defined positions and the positions detected by our tracking method. Measurements were made in pixel space and then converted to mm space using the pixel to mm ratio R_{xray} which is estimated using $R_{xray} = R_{\det} / M$. We achieved a 2D detection error of 0.5 mm ± 0.3 mm for all images and we obtained a similar error of 0.6 mm ± 0.5 mm for low dose X-ray images only.

Our method is robust in low dose images as the errors in low dose images were similar to the errors in normal dose images. Overall, we only observed detection failure in 13 frames and partial failure of detection in 14 frames. We classify a failure case if our tracking method detected the wrong catheter or other instrument and we classify a partial failure when the detection method correctly detected the ablation catheter but the method detected the wrong side of the tip head. The overall success rate of detection was 97.5%.

The major computational load of our ablation tracking method is the blob detection algorithm. We implemented it on the Intel Integrated Performance Primitives Library for fast image convolution calculation. Our method currently achieves a frame rate of 15 frames-per-second using a single-threaded CPU implementation. The performance was evaluated on an Intel Core 2 Duo 2.0GHz laptop with an nVidia Quadro FX 350M graphics card.

3.2 Motion Gating Results

To test the accuracy of the motion gating using the CS catheter, we acquired 24 sets of short biplane X-ray image sequences from 6 clinical cases. Those images were a subset of the images we tested for 2D ablation catheter tip tracking error. A pair of biplane images with the minimum reconstruction error of the proximal electrode of the CS catheter was selected using the error matrix. The motion gating error was defined as the reconstruction error of the manually defined position of the ablation catheter tip head as we tried to remove the influence of ablation catheter tip tracking errors. 0.9 mm ± 0.4 mm was achieved. Without motion gating, the reconstruction error of ablation catheter tip was 5.2 mm ± 2.9 mm. The average speed of motion gating was 650 milliseconds. This excludes the computation time of catheter tracking. As catheter tracking is real-time, it can be done while images are being acquired.

3.3 Whole System Validation

As further validation of the whole automatic tagging system, automatically detected 2D positions of ablation catheter tip head were used and the reconstruction errors of the ablation catheter tip head were computed. As the 3D positions of the ablation catheter tip head are mapped onto the surfaces of 3D roadmap, the tagging errors of the whole system have to include the registration error between the 3D roadmap and live X-ray images. We can reduce the registration errors caused by respiratory motion using real-time CS catheter tracking. In this paper, we use the same method as it was used to validate the CS catheter based motion correction method for EP procedure [13] to compute the registration errors. Finally, the whole tagging system error contains two parts. One is the motion gating error and ablation catheter tip tracking error. This can be evaluated by computing the reconstruction errors of automatically detected position of ablation catheter tip head. We calculated those errors on the same dataset used for evaluating the motion gating errors and achieved 1.1 mm ± 0.5 mm. The second part is the registration error and 1.4 mm ± 0.7 mm was achieved. The overall errors of our tagging system are difficult to compute as the exact 3D ablation positions on heart muscle are not known.

4 Conclusion and Discussions

We have developed an automatic image-based ablation point tagging system for AF ablation procedures. It is based on real-time simultaneous detection of the CS catheter and the ablation catheter. Our tracking method remains robust and accurate even in low dose fluoroscopy images as catheter electrodes remain highly visible. Our CS catheter based motion gating method significantly improves the accuracy of 3D reconstruction of the ablation catheter tip using a mono-plane X-ray system. Therefore, the tagging system can be not only used in the biplane X-ray system but also can be used in cheaper and more accessible mono-plane X-ray systems. In addition, tracking the CS catheter can be used for real-time motion correction for 3D roadmap overlay guidance. Both CS catheter tracking and ablation catheter tracking do not require any user interaction and can detect catheters without defining a region of interest in the X-ray image. For a biplane X-ray system, our tagging system is real-time. For mono-plane X-ray system, our system only requires two short image sequences and computes the 3D position on the roadmap efficiently (less than 1 second). Motion gating even could detect a failed case of ablation catheter tip detection as the large reconstruction error of the catheter tip will prevent the image being selected by the motion gating method. All these factors could lead to a widespread cost-effective alternative tagging system to commercial catheter tracking systems.

References

1. Rhode, K.S., Hill, D.L.G., Edwards, P.J., Hipwell, J., Rueckert, D., Sanchez-Ortiz, G., Hegde, S., Rahunathan, V., Razavi, R.: Registration and tracking to integrate X-ray and MR images in an XMR facility. IEEE Transactions on Medical Imaging 24(11), 810–815 (2003)
2. Hertrich, P.: Practical Radiography - Principles and Applications, 1st edn. Publicis Corporate Publishing, Erlangen (2005)
3. Pruemmer, M., Hornegger, J., Lauritsch, G., Wigstrom, L., Girard-Hughes, E., Fahrig, R.: Cardiac C-arm CT: a unified framework for motion estimation and dynamic CT. IEEE Trans. Med. Imaging 28(11), 1836–1849 (2009)
4. Orlov, M.V., Hoffmeister, P., Chaudhry, G.M., Almasry, I., Gijsbers, G.H., Swack, T., Haffajee, C.I.: Three-dimensional rotational angiography of the left atrium and esophagus– A virtual computed tomography scan in the electrophysiology lab. Heart Rhythm 4(1), 37–43 (2007)
5. Tang, M., Kriatselis, C., Ye, G., Nedios, S., Roser, M., Solowjowa, N., Fleck, E., Gerds-Li, J.H.: Reconstructing and registering three-dimensional rotational angiogram of left atrium during ablation of atrial fibrillation. Pacing Clin. Electrophysiol. 32(11), 1407–1416 (2009)
6. Knecht, S., Skali, H., O'Neill, M.D., Wright, M., Matsuo, S., Chaudhry, G.M., Haffajee, C.I., Nault, I., Gijsbers, G.H., Sacher, F., Laurent, F., Montaudon, M., Corneloup, O., Hocini, M., Haïssaguerre, M., Orlov, M.V., Jaïs, P.: Computed tomography-fluoroscopy overlay evaluation during catheter ablation of left atrial arrhythmia. Europace 10(8), 931–938 (2008)
7. Brooks, A.G., Wilson, L., Kuklik, P., Stiles, M.K., John, B., Shashidhar, D.H., Lau, D.H., Roberts-Thomson, R.L., Wong, C.X., Young, G.D., Sanders, P.: Image integration using NavX fusion: Initial experience and validation. Heart Rhythm 5(4), 526–535 (2008)
8. Franken, E., Rongen, P., van Almsick, M., ter Haar Romeny, B.M.: Detection of Electrophysiology Catheters in Noisy Fluoroscopy Images. In: Larsen, R., Nielsen, M., Sporring, J. (eds.) MICCAI 2006. LNCS, vol. 4191, pp. 25–32. Springer, Heidelberg (2006)
9. King, A.P., Boubertakh, R., Rhode, K.S., Ma, Y.L., Chinchapatnam, P., Gao, G., Tangcharoen, T., Ginks, M., Hawkes, D.J., Razavi, R.S., Schaeffter, T.: A subject-specific technique for respiratory motion correction in image-guided cardiac catheterisation procedures. Med. Image. Anal. 13(3), 419–431 (2009)

10. Shechter, G., Shechter, B., Resar, J.R., Beyar, R.: Prospective motion correction of X-ray images for coronary interventions. IEEE Transactions on Medical Imaging 24(4), 441–450 (2005)
11. Sundar, H., Khamene, A., Yatziv, L., Xu, C.: Automatic Image-Based Cardiac and Respiratory Cycle Synchronization and Gating of Image Sequences. In: Yang, G.-Z., Hawkes, D., Rueckert, D., Noble, A., Taylor, C. (eds.) MICCAI 2009. LNCS, vol. 5762, pp. 381–388. Springer, Heidelberg (2009)
12. Brost, A., Liao, R., Strobel, N., Hornegger, J.: Respiratory motion compensation by model-based catheter tracking during EP procedures. Med. Image. Anal. 14(5), 695–706 (2010)
13. Ma, Y., King, A.P., Gogin, N., Rinaldi, C.A., Gill, J., Razavi, R., Rhode, K.S.: Real-time respiratory motion correction for cardiac electrophysiology procedures using image-based coronary sinus catheter tracking. In: Jiang, T., Navab, N., Pluim, J.P.W., Viergever, M.A. (eds.) MICCAI 2010. LNCS, vol. 6361, pp. 391–399. Springer, Heidelberg (2010)
14. Hoffman, K., Sen, A., Lan, L., Metz, C., Chua, K., Williams, B., Esthappen, J., Fiebich, M., Mazzucco, M., Doi, K.: Determination of 3-D vessel trees from biplane images from coronary angiography. Computer. Assisted Radiology Surgery, 162–165 (1997)
15. Tony, L.: Detecting salient blob-like image structures and their scales with a scale-space primal sketch: a Method for focus-of-attention. International Journal of Computer Vision 11(3), 283–318 (1993)

Passive Single Marker Tracking for Organ Motion and Deformation Detection in Open Liver Surgery

Thiago Oliveira-Santos*, Matthias Peterhans, Simon Hofmann, and Stefan Weber

ARTORG Center for Computer Aided Surgery, University of Bern, Switzerland
thiago.oliveira@istb.unibe.ch

Abstract. Organ motion and deformation are major obstacles hindering the introduction of image guidance into soft tissue surgery. Due to challenges with update rate, invasiveness and intra-operative complexity, there is currently no clinically established solution for deformation measurements on soft tissues. We present a soft tissue tracking approach based on single passive markers as part of a navigation system for open liver surgery. Such markers are minimally-invasive and allow for real-time organ motion measurements using available tracking systems. The absence of correspondence between position measurements over time and the sensitivity to other reflectors present within the workspace inhibit the direct clinical implementation of such technology. Hence, we remove measurement artifacts, establish marker correspondence over time, and achieve robustness against occlusions and presence of other reflecting objects. A thorough experimental evaluation demonstrates reliable motion tracking and motivates its use for deformation detection and respiratory gating in open liver surgery.

Keywords: Liver Surgery, Image Guided Surgery, Soft Tissue Tracking, Fiducial Marker Tracking.

1 Introduction

Computer assistance through surgical navigation systems has been applied in many surgical domains, such as orthopaedic-, neuro-, and ENT (i.e. ear, nose and throat) surgery [1], [2], [3]. With these systems, pre-operative planning data can be co-displayed in a registered virtual context providing surgeons with intra-operative instrument guidance. The motion of rigid anatomical structures (e.g. bone, head) can be easily tracked by means of an attached dynamic reference base (DRB). Soft tissue structures, however, deform significantly during surgical interventions and this deformation cannot be detected or represented by the attachment of a DRB.

To address this problem, Vetter *et al.*, [4], used electro-magnetic position measurement devices to determine the position of navigation aids anchored to the liver in order to monitor possible liver deformations. Such electro-magnetic technology, although suitable for biopsies and ablation scenarios, may be very sensitive to ferromagnetic material present in open surgeries. With a similar approach, Maier-Hein *et al.*, [5], [6],

* Corresponding author.

R.H. Taylor and G.-Z. Yang (Eds.): IPCAI 2011, LNCS 6689, pp. 156–167, 2011.

[7], proposed the use of optical position measurement devices to track needles placed in the liver and to estimate the deformation around the target. Their ex-vivo results [5] show the technique copes well with deformations present in CT-guided minimally invasive interventions. However, its applicability in a scenario where the liver is manually handled and deformed, as in open liver surgery, was not evaluated. Using a video based tracking system, Nicolau *et al.* proposed [8], [9], [10] methods for tracking and registering a radio-opaque marker set attached to the patient skin. With such techniques, soft tissue tracking can be achieved and used for radio frequency hepatic tumor ablation [8]. With a more complex setup, Cash *et al.* [11], [12] integrated a laser range scanner intra-operatively in order to digitize the exposed liver surface. The intra-operative data was then registered with the pre-operative model and a finite element approach was used to account for organ deformations. By means of available tracking systems, Markert *et al.* [13] proposed a method to track and estimate liver deformation during open surgery based on a retro-reflective single marker (SM) set placed on the liver surface. The position of each SM is detected with an optical tracking system and the liver position and deformation is estimated. The results demonstrated the feasibility of calculating the position of points on the liver surface using a SM set. Nevertheless, the robustness of the tracking algorithm was not evaluated in the study. Due to challenges with update rate, invasiveness and intra-operative complexity, there is currently no clinically established solution for soft tissue tracking.

In this work, we propose a solution to track deformable structures (e.g. liver) based on retro-reflective SMs. The differences to [13] lie in the strong focus on clinical usability and in the detailed description of a scalable and fast implementation of SM tracking using readily available position measurement systems. Such markers are minimally-invasive and allow for real-time measurement of organ surface motion while using available passive optical tracking systems. Two main disadvantages associated with this tracking technology are addressed in this work: the presence of phantom positions (i.e. position of markers not really present in the scene) and the lack of correspondence between SM positions across different tracking frames. The robustness of our SM tracking algorithm against different conditions that might be faced in the Operating Room (OR) is assessed in a lab setup. As the tracking system used to track the instruments and the organ is the same, the algorithm should handle: deformation of the organ, the presence of unexpected markers and other instruments as well as recover from partial and total occlusions. The use of pair-point rigid registration for deformation detection is also investigated. In addition, a workflow for clinical integration of the SM tracking in open liver surgery is presented.

2 Materials and Method

The proposed solution relies on data provided by a NDI Vicra (Northern Digital Inc., Waterloo, Canada) position measurement system (*pms*) which tracks a set of SMs attached to the surface of an organ. Each SM comprises a retro-reflective sphere fixed to a post which is attached directly to a soft organ. The Vicra *pms* is configured to supply data containing the pose of each tracked DRB, plus any detected position of stray markers that are reflected in the scene and do not belong to a tracked DRB, i.e. ${}^{pms}P_{STR}$. The Vicra *pms* works as a black box that returns the transformations of the detected DRBs and positions of the detected stray markers without providing real time access to the captured images. Therefore, any possible image processing (segmentation, rectification, etc) is performed internally and is not accessible during tracking. The SM tracking algorithm uses the data supplied by the Vicra to estimate the organ (*org*) pose, i.e. the rigid transformation ${}^{pms}T_{org}$ from *org* to *pms*, as well as a set of vectors, i.e. ${}^{org}V_{SM}$, representing the deformation of the SMs in the organ (see **Fig. 1**).

As mentioned before, ${}^{pms}P_{STR}$ requires special handling. Firstly, phantom positions are removed. These occur when the Vicra cannot find a unique correspondence between the detected markers in both sensor images. The ambiguity appears whenever two or more markers reflecting in the scene share the same epipolar line. Theoretically, the number of phantom positions increases with the number of SMs meeting these conditions, i.e. *n* SMs in the same epipolar line would create up to $n.(n\text{-}1)$ phantom positions. Therefore, the set of positions ${}^{pms}P_{STR}$ includes not only the SM positions in the viewing volume, but also all phantom positions created according to the criteria above. Once phantom markers are removed, the correspondence between SMs of different frames needs to be established. As the *pms* relies only on information of the current frame to estimate the 3D position of a marker, the same SM on the organ surface might have a different indexes (i.e. labels) in the set of positions ${}^{pms}P_{STR}$ of different frames.

In order to evaluate the proposed solution, a navigation system [14] developed to assist open liver surgery was augmented with the SM tracking algorithm and used in our experiments.

2.1 SM Tracking Algorithm

The tracking algorithm is based on the assumptions that a non-symmetrical SM placement is chosen (e.g. not a regular grid) and that an initial configuration, i.e. the initial SM positions ${}^{org}P_{SM*}$ in the organ coordinate system, can be defined. The positions ${}^{org}P_{SM*}$ represent a tracking state without deformation. The actual SM tracking algorithm comprises 5 modules (see **Fig. 1** right): **1. Phantom Removal**: is continuously applied to ${}^{pms}P_{STR}$ in order to create a phantoms free set of positions, i.e. ${}^{pms}P_{PHF}$; **2. Initial Configuration Definition**: is performed once, prior to the commencement of SM tracking in order to define ${}^{org}P_{SM*}$; **3. SM Re-Labeling**: is performed at each frame to find the current corresponding SM positions ${}^{pms}P_{SM}$ in ${}^{pms}P_{PHF}$; **4. Geometrical Checking**: ensures ${}^{pms}P_{SM}$ respects the geometrical constraints set by ${}^{org}P_{SM*}$; **5. Pose & Deformation Estimation**: calculates ${}^{pms}T_{org}$ and ${}^{org}V_{SM}$ based on ${}^{pms}P_{SM}$ and ${}^{org}P_{SM*}$.

1. Phantom Removal. The SMs are assumed to lie at a similar distance to the *pms* (i.e. with the liver surface is oriented perpendicularly to the *pms*). Therefore, this module treats the situation where SMs lie more or less in plane perpendicular to the *pms* depth direction (z-axis), illustrated in **Fig. 2 b,** and disregards alternative situations illustrated in **Fig. 2 a** (configurations with one SM behind another from the *pms* point of view). The module relies on the CCD sensor locations within the stereoscopic *pms*, ${}^{pms}P_{S1}$ and ${}^{pms}P_{S2}$ (see **Fig. 3**), to identify and remove the phantom positions.

For every frame, a line connecting each position measurement in ${}^{pms}P_{STR}$ and the *pms* origin is calculated. The intersection between these lines and a plane (defined in front of the sensors and with normal pointing to *pms* z direction, see **Fig. 2**) generates a set of corresponding intersection points ${}^{pms}P_{STR}'$. A phantom position $C \in {}^{pms}P_{STR}$ is likely to be generated whenever two real positions, A and $B \in {}^{pms}P_{STR}$, have their corresponding A' and $B' \in {}^{pms}P_{STR}'$ with similar x values (within a tolerance of 5mm that was empirically chosen to capture all phantoms generated within the viewing volume of the *pms*). C is considered a phantom candidate whenever the x component of the corresponding C' has a similar value to A' or B'. Every position in ${}^{pms}P_{STR}$ has a confidence measure for being a real SM and another confidence measure for being a phantom. The confidence measure for the positions A and B to be real SMs and the position C to be a phantom are incremented by one every time the lines passing through (A,B), (B,C), and (C,A), i.e. $L_{(A,B)}$, $L_{(B,C)}$ and $L_{(C,A)}$ respectively, meet the following requirements: $L_{(A,B)}$ crosses the camera sensor plane in the *pms*'s lateral region and each of $L_{(B,C)}$ and $L_{(C,A)}$ crosses the camera sensor plane in one of the sensor regions (see **Fig. 3** for the definition of the regions). After evaluating all positions, the those with higher confidence measures for being real than for being phantom are assigned to the set of filtered positions ${}^{pms}P_{PHF}$. This approach eliminates phantom positions of up to two SMs sharing the same epipolar line, however it cannot remove all whenever more than two SMs meet this condition. In order to eliminate the remaining phantom positions when three SMs share the same epipolar line, the procedure described above is applied a second time to ${}^{pms}P_{PHF}$.

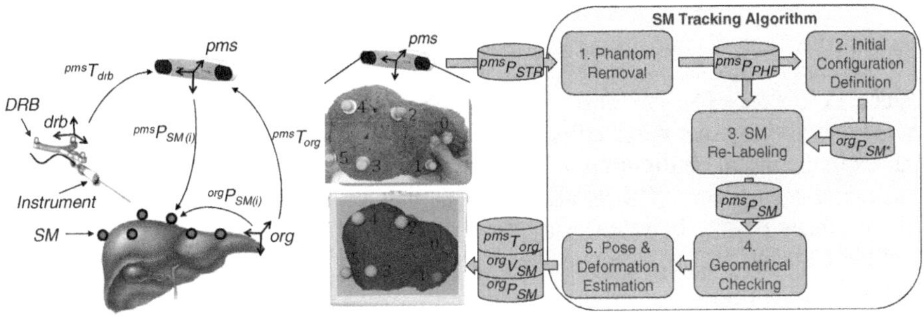

Fig. 1. Illustration of the coordinate systems and transformations (left). Illustration of the data flow within the SM tracking algorithm (right).

2. Initial Configuration Definition. The SM configuration, ${}^{pms}P_{PHF}$, at the start of the tracking algorithm is assigned to ${}^{org}P_{SM*}$. This initial arrangement specifies a local coordinate system *org* to the tracked organ, defines a label for each SM, and imposes the geometrical constraints between them.

3. SM Re-Labeling. To re-label the positions in the current frame ${}^{pms}P_{PHF}$ according to ${}^{org}P_{SM*}$, two methods are used: *distance based labeling* and *previous-frame based labeling*. In order to give preference to the initial configuration spatial arrangement, the former is tried first and in case of failure, the latter is used.

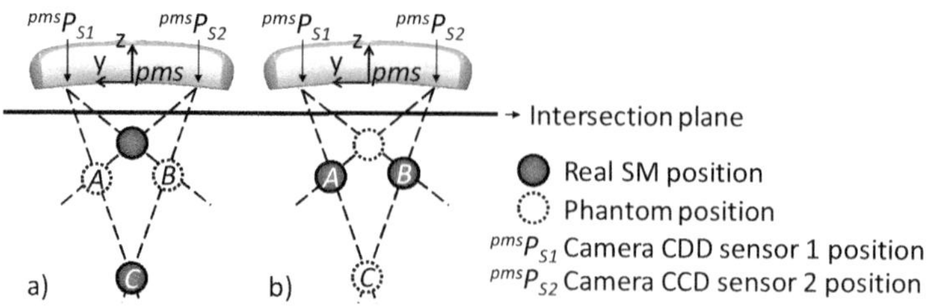

Fig. 2. Illustration of two situations, **a)** and **b)**, where phantom markers are created

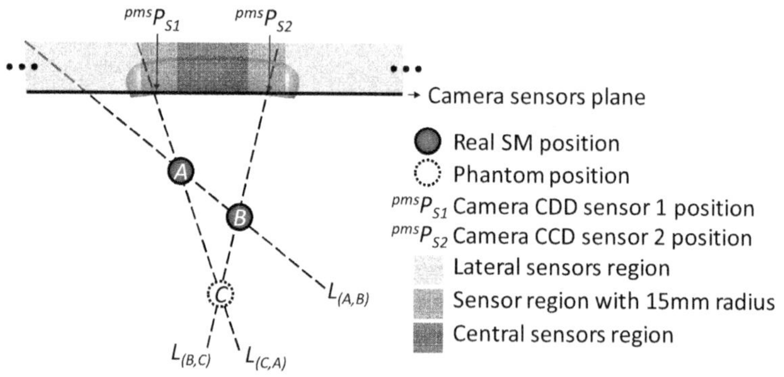

Fig. 3. Illustration of the phantom removal

The *distance based labeling* requires that all SMs are visible and therefore contained in $^{pms}P_{PHF}$. The labeling compares the distances between a position to be labeled and all the other detected positions with the possible sets of corresponding distances in the initial configuration. The label is finally assigned to the position with the most similar distances. The similarity is calculated through a cost function based on the distances $D_{SM*(i,j)}$ between every pair of SMs in the initial configuration $^{pms}P_{SM*}$, and the distances $D_{PHF(m,n)}$ between every pair of current measured positions $^{pms}P_{PHF}$, as follows:

$$c\_2_{(a,b,c,d)} = \sum_{m \neq a, m \neq c}^{M} min_{n \neq b, n \neq d}^{N}(|D_{SM*(a,m)} - D_{PHF(b,n)}|) \quad (1)$$

$$c\_1_{(i,j)} = \sum_{m \neq i}^{M} (min_{n \neq j}^{N}(|D_{SM*(i,m)} - D_{PHF(j,n)}|) + c\_2_{(m,n,i,j)}) \quad (2)$$

$$n\_c\_1_{(i,j)} = \frac{c\_1_{(i,j)}}{\sum_{m}^{M} c\_1_{(i,m)}} \quad (3)$$

where, M and N are the number of elements in $^{pms}P_{SM*}$ and $^{pms}P_{PHF}$ respectively. The functions *c_1*, c_2 and *n_c_1* calculate the cost of position j to correspond to a label i. The cost is represented by the sum of the differences between the distance of the searched i and each of the remaining SMs in the initial configuration $^{pms}P_{SM*}$ and the most similar distance between the searched *j* and the remaining positions in the current detected positions ${}^{pms}P_{PHF}$. While c_1 calculates the cost of the distances in the first level (from the evaluated *i* to the remaining positions *n*), c_2 adds a second level of confidence by considering the distances from the position *n* (selected in c_1 as the best distance to *i*) to the remaining positions. The addition of c_2 makes the tracking more robust to ambiguous assignments. Finally, the function n_c_1 normalizes the cost to ensure that positions with significantly smaller cost values for a certain label have higher priority. Subsequently, an exhaustive search finds the pair *(a, b)* with the minimum value in n_c_1 and the position ${}^{pms}P_{PHF(a)}$ is assigned to ${}^{pms}P_{SM(b)}$.

Two additional terms are evaluated while assigning a position to an SM. Firstly, the difference between the distances in ${}^{pms}P_{SM}$ and the respective distances in ${}^{pms}P_{SM^*}$ should be within a threshold (an empirical value of 40mm was chosen to safely allow for organ deformation that is consistent with the literature [15]). Secondly, the new position should not differ excessively from its corresponding position in the previous frame if it was visible (an empirical limit of 30mm was chosen based on a maximum speed of the surgical actions and the update rate of the *pms*). The first factor limits the amount of deformation allowed, whereas the second gives priority to positions more similar to the SM location in the previous frame.

In *previous-frame based labeling*, the current position of each SM ${}^{pms}P_{SM(i)}$ is updated to the closest position in ${}^{pms}P_{PHF}$, as follow:

$$\text{If } {}^{pms}P_{SM(i)} \text{ was visible, } {}^{pms}P_{SM(i)} = closest({}^{pms}P_{SM(i)}, {}^{pms}P_{PHF}) \tag{4}$$

$$\text{If } {}^{pms}P_{SM(i)} \text{ was invisible, } {}^{pms}P_{SM(i)} = closest({}^{pms}T_{org} \cdot {}^{org}P_{SM^*(i)}, {}^{pms}P_{PHF}) \tag{5}$$

where, $closest(P_{(i)},P_{PHF})$ returns the position in P_{PHF} that is the closest to $P_{(i)}$ within a radius (set to 30mm as above); and, ${}^{pms}T_{org}$ is the previous pose of the organ. In cases where there is no position within the defined radius, the SM is set to invisible.

4. Geometrical Checking. This module ensures that at least a minimum number (set to 4 in this study) of SMs are visible, and that the distances between the new SM positions are still below a tolerance $Threshold_{dist}$. The check is performed by comparing the distances between every two subsequent visible SMs and the corresponding distance in the initial configuration, as below:

$$|D_{SM(i,\,mod((i+1),\,M))} - D_{SM^*((i,\,mod((i+1),\,M)))}| < Threshold_{dist} = 40\text{mm} \tag{6}$$

In case of failure, the organ is set to invisible.

5. Pose & Deformation Estimation. In this module, the pose ${}^{pms}T_{org}$ is estimated by minimizing the square distances between SM positions in ${}^{org}P_{SM^*}$ and their corresponding positions in ${}^{pms}P_{SM}$, as proposed in [16]. The deformation represented by fiducial registration error is then calculated as:

$${}^{org}V_{SM} = {}^{org}P_{SM^*} - {}^{pms}T_{org}^{-1} \cdot {}^{pms}P_{SM} \tag{7}$$

2.2 Surgical Workflow

The surgical workflow is divided into 4 steps illustrated in **Fig. 4**.

1. Planning. The surgical planning is performed pre-operatively based on a CT dataset. The liver is segmented (using MeVis Distant Services, Germany) to generate a 3D model that is uploaded to the navigation system prior to surgery.

2. Surgical Setup. Once the liver is stable, the SM set is attached to the organ surface with biocompatible cyanoacrylate glue [17] (tested on ex-vivo liver). A total of six SMs are placed (mostly in the area to be resected) in order to keep a good tradeoff between organ representation and the remaining working space for the surgical intervention.

3. Registration. Once the SM set is in place, the surgeon performs a registration of the real liver to its virtual 3D model. The point-wise registration between the 3D model and the real liver is accomplished using liver anatomical landmarks. Alternatively, other more advanced methods such as ultrasound based registration could be used. At this point, the initial configuration is defined.

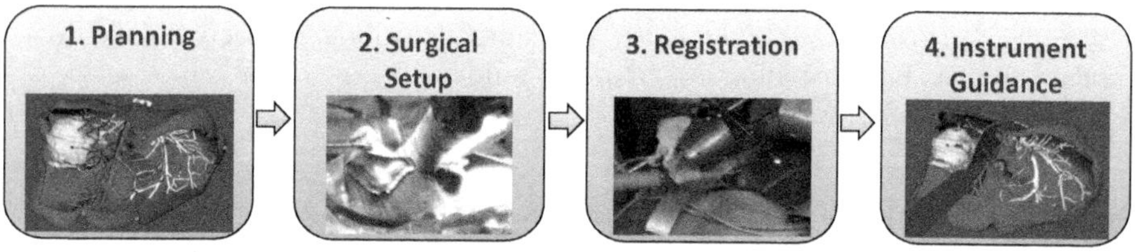

Fig. 4. Surgical workflow overview

4. Instrument Guidance. After the initial setup, the 3D model of the liver is co-displayed with the other tracked instruments. A color coding is used to represent the deformation, $|^{org}V_{SM(i)}|$, of each SM (see **Fig. 1** right). The surgeon uses the deformation information provided by the system to identify an optimal tracking situation, i.e. where the deformation from the initial configuration is minimal.

2.3 Evaluation Experiments

A set of experiments was performed to validate the presented approach.

Organ Tracking. A silicon liver was tracked by means of six SMs attached to its surface in different arrangements. Firstly, the liver was rotated in front of the position measurement system five times (each with a different SM set arrangement) by 360° so that phantom positions were produced (see **Fig. 5a**). The rate of phantom positions produced and the efficiency of the phantom removal were measured. In a second step, the silicon liver was tracked 10 times (each with a different SM set arrangement) while evaluating different scenarios (see **Table 1**). A scenario was considered problematic for an arrangement if there was an error *ERR* (i.e. wrong markers assignment) at any point during tracking. The percentage of arrangements with error for each scenario was then calculated. Additionally, the processing time for the SM tracking algorithm was assessed while tracking different number of SMs.

Pose Estimation. To validate whether the liver pose estimated with the SM is comparable to its pose estimated with a DRB in an optimal rigid scenario, a rigid liver was tracked by means of six SMs as well as by a DRB. Four target points in the liver surface were defined relative to the DRB ${}^{drb}P_{TAR}$ and relative to the tracked organ ${}^{org}P_{TAR}$. The liver was systematically moved up and down, as well as rotated in two axes (**Fig. 5d**). The target registration error *TRE* of these points was measured for each tracked frame using the following:

$$TRE_i = | {}^{drb}P_{TAR(i)} - {}^{pms}T_{drb}{}^{-1} \cdot {}^{pms}T_{org} \cdot {}^{org}P_{TAR(i)} | \tag{8}$$

Deformation Identification. To show that deformation of the tracked organ can be identified, a set of seven SMs were attached to the silicon liver. One SM was used as target ${}^{pms}P_{TAR}$, whereas the remaining six were used for organ tracking. The liver was then tracked under two different scenarios illustrated in **Fig. 5b** and **c** (representing diaphragm and handling respectively). The changes of ${}^{pms}P_{TAR}$ (i.e. distance from its current position to its position at the time of the initial configuration definition) were continuously measured and compared to the changes in the average deformation value $|\overline{{}^{org}V_{SM}}|$.

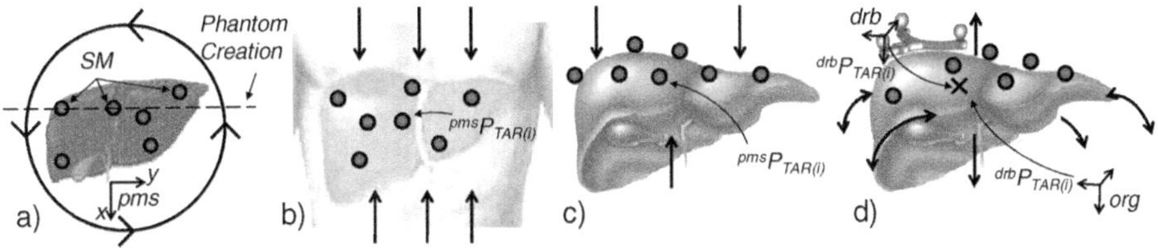

Fig. 5. a) Phantom experiment: arrows represent the liver rotation. **b)** Axial compression: arrows represent the direction of forces applied. **c)** Handling: arrows represent the direction of forces applied. **d)** Rigid motion: arrows represent the direction of motion. Target point is represented by the x.

3 Results and Discussion

Organ Tracking. The results of the first experiment in **Fig. 6a** show that phantom positions are quite often produced by the Vicra *pms*. It can be seen that roughly one peak is obtained for any angle where one pair or three markers are coplanar with the camera centers. For all five arrangements tested, phantom positions were present in 15% (average) of the cases while rotating the liver by 360° (1, 2, 3 and 4 phantom positions were produced in 6%, 8.5%, 0.3% and 0.2% of the cases respectively). Further analyses of the ${}^{pms}P_{PHF}$ generated during these experiments showed that the phantom removal algorithm efficiently eliminated all phantom positions produced. The results of tracking under different scenarios, presented in **Table 2**, show the SM tracking was robust enough to handle most of them when tracking 10 different SM arrangements. The results of the processing time experiment show that the complete SM tracking algorithm performs in 1.17, 5.01, 9.75, 12.82 and 22.84ms for 6, 7, 8, 9 and 10 SMs defining the organ respectively (on an Intel Core 2 Quad 3GHz with 4G RAM).

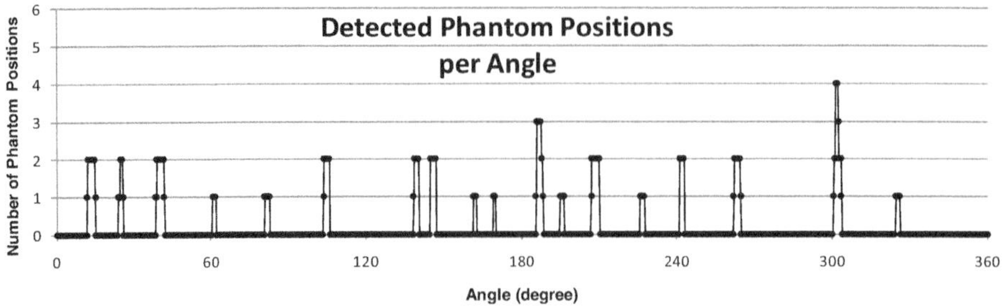

Fig. 6. Frequency of phantom positions produced during one 360° rotation of the liver in front of the *pms* for one of the SM set arrangements

Table 1. Scenarios applied during tracking

M_{RIG}	Rigid Motion	Liver was moved in front of the Vicra
DEF	Deformation	Liver was deformed as illustrated in **Fig. 5b** and **c**
OCC_{PAR}	Partial occlusion	Liver was partially occluded considering different SMs
OCC_{TOT}	Total occlusion	Liver was totally occluded from different sides
UR	Unexpected reflection	Four extra SMs were added to the scene
DRB	Presence of a DRB	DRB placed between the camera and the SMs

Table 2. Percentage of errors (i.e. wrong marker assignments) for 10 different SM arrangements under different tracking scenarios

Scenario	***ERR* (%)**	***ERR* (%) per Scenarios Combination**					
		M_{RIG}	*DEF*	OCC_{PAR}	OCC_{TOT}	*UR*	**DRBs**
M_{RIG}	0		0	0	0		
DEF	10			0	0		0
OCC_{PAR}	0					10	0
OCC_{TOT}	0					100	0
UR	100						
DRBs	0						

In the scenario *UR*, tracking was mostly stable whilst moving the extra SM in the scene. Errors occurred in 100% of the arrangements when one extra SM was close (less than 50mm) to one of the SMs on the organ and between its line-of-sight with the Vicra. In this case, the extra SM took over the label of the covered organ marker. Nonetheless, the label was again correctly assigned as soon as the extra maker stopped occluding the SM on the organ, and therefore was not considered a major concern. In the scenario combination $UR + OCC_{TOT}$, errors were also present in 100% of the cases when recovering from a total occlusion with extra SMs continuously placed close to the SMs on the organ. The extra SMs assumed the label of some of the organ SMs which were still occluded and the correct label assignment could only be recovered after occluding the extra SMs. However, this is not expected to happen very often in the OR and can be avoided by identifying and covering the unexpected reflections in the scene. The same case also occurred with partial occlusion of the organ SMs (scenario combination $UR + OCC_{TOT}$), but only for one arrangement. Confusion of the organ SMs with the DRB geometries defined in the position measurement system occurred for one SM arrangement while deforming the liver (scenario *DEF*). However, it only caused the organ to be invisible for a few milliseconds because the respective SMs could not be detected by the position measurement system in this case. This situation as well as possible wrong label assignment due to bad SM arrangement choice, can be avoided by providing position profiles to the surgeon. Such profiles can guide the surgeon roughly during the SM attachment in order to have a pre-optimized SM arrangement.

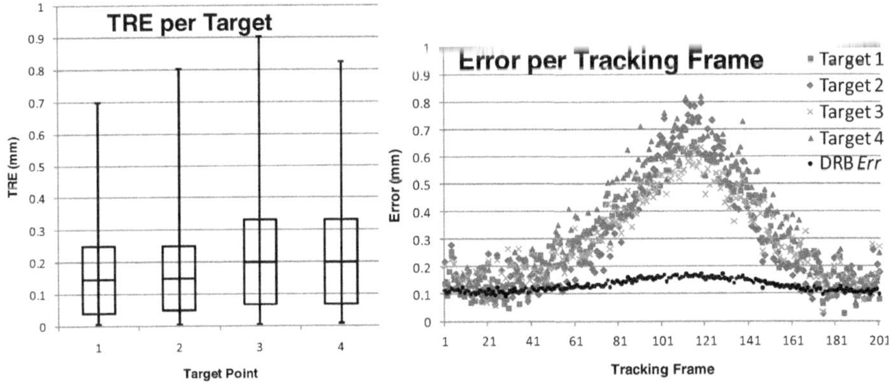

Fig. 7. (Left) Boxplot of TRE values for the 4 targets for 5 SM arrangements. (Right) Difference in target localization and DRB fitting error for one of the SM arrangement.

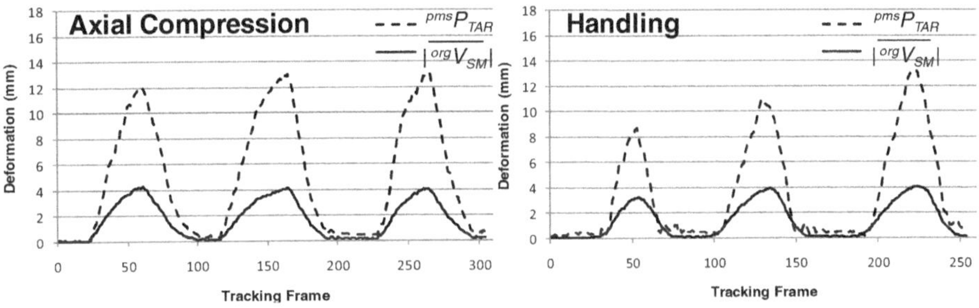

Fig. 8. Comparison of deformation measured by single markers and one evaluation point under axial compression and simulated surgical handling of a silicon liver phantom

Pose Estimation. The results in **Fig. 7** left show that the average differences in the localization of 4 target points by a rigid DRB and by a set of SMs are below 0.2mm. The maximal differences of 0.9mm could be attributed to tracking errors (i.e. fitting error to the pre-defined geometry) on both, the DRB (*DRB Err*) and the SMs (*SMs err*). These errors are not correlated with each other (correlation value of 0.2), but are correlated with the TRE of the target points on the organ (correlation values of 0.6 and 0.59 respectively). **Fig. 7** right illustrates the correlation between the TREs and the *DRB Err* and shows how the localization error is propagated to the targets.

Dleformation Identification. The curves in **Fig. 8** show a comparison between deformation measurements obtained from averaging the SM errors and the local motion measurement on a single point of the silicon phantom. The strong correlation of 0.98 and 0.96 between the two curves in **Fig. 8.a** and **b** respectively indicates that organ deformation can be reliably detected using SMs.

4 Conclusions

This paper presents an approach for soft tissue tracking based on passive single markers attached to an organ surface that are tracked by an optical sensor. Our experiments demonstrated that our approach is capable of tracking deformable organs, such as the liver, in real time and under different constraints, representing real OR conditions. It was also demonstrated, that a tracking accuracy, comparable to rigid reference bases (i.e. tracker) could be achieved throughout real world conditions. The evaluation scenarios were chosen with focus on the clinical application and considering the experience gained in previous navigated liver surgeries [14]. Additionally, tracking of a soft organ using single optical markers allows for precise detection of its deformation state. Although, deformation of the soft organ can be detected using the described approach its compensation must still be addressed in the future. An algorithm is described to identify false positive phantom markers that are detected by the optical tracking system. These phantom markers are successfully neglected throughout the further processing of the tracking information. To cope with the dynamic OR environment, our approach can recover from occlusions of some or even all the single markers. A main advantage is the possibility to combine single markers and rigid references together in one workspace, allowing for a simultaneous tracking of instruments and the organ in real time.

Although this approach to soft tissue tracking was evaluated only under laboratory conditions, we believe that it will be possible to transfer into a clinical environment and ultimately deploy in computer-assisted liver surgery.

References

1. Taylor, R.H., Lavallée, S., et al.: Computer-Integrated Surgery: Technology and Clinical Applications. MIT Press, Cambridge (1995)
2. Peters, T.M.: Image-guidance for surgical procedures. Phys. Med. Biol. 51(14), R505-R540 (2006)
3. Yaniv, Z., Cleary, K.: Image-guided procedures: A review. Technical report, Georgetown University (2006)
4. Vetter, M., Wolf, I., et al.: Navigation aids and real-time deformation modeling for open liver surgery. In: Proceedings of the SPIE, vol. 5029, pp. 58–68 (2003)
5. Maier-Hein, L., Maleike, D., et al.: Soft tissue navigation using needle-shaped markers: Evaluation of navigation aid tracking accuracy and CT registration. In: Proceedings of the SPIE 2007, vol. 6509, p. 26 (2007)
6. Maier-Hein, L., Tekbas, A., et al.: In vivo accuracy assessment of a needle-based navigation system for CT-guided radiofrequency ablation of the liver. Med. Phys. 35(12), 5385–5396 (2008)

7. Maier-Hein, L., Tekbas, A., et al.: On combining internal and external fiducials for liver motion compensation. Comp. Aid Surg. 13(16), 369–376 (2008)
8. Nicolau, S., Garcia, A., et al.: An augmented reality system to guide radio-frequency tumor ablation. Computer Animation and Virtual World 16(1), 1–10 (2005)
9. Nicolau, S.A., Pennec, X., Soler, L., Ayache, N.: Clinical evaluation of a respiratory gated guidance system for liver punctures. In: Ayache, N., Ourselin, S., Maeder, A. (eds.) MICCAI 2007, Part II. LNCS, vol. 4792, pp. 77–85. Springer, Heidelberg (2007)
10. Nicolau, S.A., Pennec, X., et al.: An augmented reality system for liver thermal ablation: design and evaluation on clinical cases. Med. Image Anal. 13(3), 494–506 (2009)
11. Cash, D.M., Miga, M.I., et al.: Compensating for intraoperative soft-tissue deformations using incomplete surface data and finite elements. IEEE T. Med. Imaging 24(11), 1479–1491 (2005)
12. Cash, D.M., Miga, M.I., et al.: Concepts and preliminary data toward the realization of image-guided liver surgery. J. Gastrointest Surg. 11(7), 844–859 (2007)
13. Markert, M., Koschany, A., Lueth, T.: Tracking of the liver for navigation in open surgery. Int. J. CARS 5, 229–235 (2010)
14. Peterhans, M., Vom Berg, A., et al.: A navigation system for open liver surgery: design, workflow and first clinical applications. Int. J. Med. Robot (2010)
15. Herline, A.J., Stefansic, J.D., et al.: Image-guided surgery: preliminary feasibility studies of frameless stereotactic liver surgery. Arch. Surg. 134(6), 644–649, discussion 649–650 (1999)
16. Veldpaus, F.E., Woltring, H.J., Dortmans, L.J.: A least-squares algorithm for the equiform transformation from spatial marker co-ordinates. J. Biomech. 21(1), 45–54 (1988)
17. Dalvi, A., Faria, M., Pinto, A.: Non-suture closure of wound using cyanoacrylate. J. Postgrad Med. 32(2), 97–100 (1986)

Improved Neuronavigation through Integration of Intraoperative Anatomical and Diffusion Images in an Interventional MRI Suite

Pankaj Daga[1], Gavin Winston[2], Marc Modat[1], M. Jorge Cardoso[1], Mark White[3], Laura Mancini[3], Andrew W. McEvoy[3], John Thornton[3], Caroline Micallef[3], Tarek Yousry[3], David Hawkes[1], John S. Duncan[2], and Sebastien Ourselin[1]

[1] Centre for Medical Image Computing (CMIC), University College London, UK
[2] Epilepsy Society MRI Unit and Department of Clinical and Experimental Epilepsy, UCL Institute of Neurology, London, UK
[3] National Hospital for Neurology and Neurosurgery, UCLH NHS Foundation Trust, London, UK

Abstract. Integration of information from complementary imaging modalities in medical image registration schemes potentially improves the registration accuracy. MRI is now being used for guidance of various neurosurgical procedures like anterior temporal lobe resection in patients with refractory temporal lobe epilepsy. Accurate localisation of critical white matter tracts, such as the optic radiation, during neurosurgery is critical in ensuring good patient outcome. Current commercial interventional MR scanners are capable of performing anatomical and diffusion weighted imaging. We propose a near real-time multivariate registration scheme that uses both anatomical and diffusion images from the pre and intraoperative imaging sessions. The registration framework is optimized for use on graphical processing units and we perform a full multivariate non-rigid registration in under three minutes making the proposed framework suitable for use under the stringent time constraints of neurosurgical procedures. We assess the accuracy of our algorithm using a numerical phantom and demonstrate accurate localisation of the optic radiation in clinical datasets. This work could be of significant utility in image guided interventions and facilitate effective surgical treatments.

1 Introduction

Neurosurgery plays an important role in the management of refractory epilepsy. Around one-third of patients with focal epilepsy are refractory to treatment with anti-epileptic drugs. Anterior temporal lobe resection is an effective treatment in such patients with refractory temporal lobe epilepsy [1]. For neurosurgical procedures, a careful balance has to be struck for each individual patient between removing the seizure focus and causing new morbidity. New morbidity can typically occur because of damage to brain areas responsible for specific functions due to the surgical intervention. An important source of morbidity

R.H. Taylor and G.-Z. Yang (Eds.): IPCAI 2011, LNCS 6689, pp. 168–178, 2011.

during anterior temporal lobe resection arises due to the damage to the optic radiation during intervention which can lead to severe visual field deficits (VFD) that can preclude a patient from driving, even if seizure free. These deficits are typically caused by damage to Meyer's loop, the most anterior part of the optic radiation, which shows considerable variability between patients in its location [2]. Hence, accurate localisation of the optic radiation during surgery is crucial in improving the surgical outcome for patients undergoing temporal lobe resection. White matter tracts, like the optic radiation, are not visible on conventional structural magnetic resonance (MR) images and require diffusion tensor imaging (DTI) and probabilistic tractography for accurate parcellation. In addition, it is also important to track anatomical structures of interest to allow surgeons to navigate during surgery using anatomical and target landmarks. Hence, image guided surgical systems that use fused information from both anatomical and diffusion images may facilitate more effective surgical treatments.

Even though current commercial interventional MR (iMR) scanners can acquire diffusion weighted (DW) images, it is not feasible to perform probabilistic tractography of the optic radiation on interventional data within the time-frame of the surgical procedure. This is due to the computational time required with current implementations of probabilistic tractography and because it requires expert user interaction in terms of placement of seed points and needs higher quality DW images to produce reliable results. A feasible solution is to use non-rigid registration to propagate the parcellated optic radiation from the preoperative to intraoperative space.

Archip *et al* [3] demonstrated a neurosurgery system capable of performing non-rigid registration and visualising imaging data from various modalities. However, it does not exploit the shared information present in the images to drive the registration. The current state-of-the-art commercial neuronavigation systems do not perform a non-rigid mapping between the pre and intraoperative images due to the computational complexity of non-rigid algorithms. In addition, the similarity measure used by these systems in the registration algorithm does not exploit the shared information that might be present between the different images. Hence, the current systems are unable to utilise the full information that is made available through the use of iMR imaging. These two factors limit the effectiveness of these systems in accurate localisation of target and eloquent brain areas.

There is relatively little work on the topic of multivariate image registration. Park *et al* [4] presented a multi-channel variation of the demons algorithm to register DTI datasets and create a group diffusion tensor atlas. Similarly, Avants *et al* [5] presented a multivariate approach using fused structural and diffusion data. Even though both these works used images from various modalities, there is no explicit formulation to utilise the shared information present in the various images. Studholme [6] introduced a novel multivariate mutual information (MI) based similarity measure called diffusion paired MI which uses structural MR and DT images in a unified similarity measure. The method uses the full tensor information and requires computation of 7 four dimensional joint histograms.

This computational complexity renders it unsuitable for use in a neurosurgical setting due to the time time constraints.

This paper extends our previous work [7] that integrated anatomical and diffusion images in a multivariate normalised mutual information (NMI) based registration similarity measure. We make the proposed registration framework suitable to be used within the time constraints of a neurosurgical procedure by exploiting the parallel processing capabilities of graphical processing units (GPU) and demonstrate its use on interventional datasets. We present the design of a surgical workflow that could benefit from this registration framework.

2 Interventional Imaging Workflow

The iMR setup at the National Hospital for Neurology and Neurosurgery (NHNN) in London consists of a 1.5T Siemens Espree MRI machine. There is a dedicated operating room 12 channel MR head coil which incorporates a surgical headrest. The operating table is fitted with a MR compatible head-holder and is placed outside the 5 Gauss line during surgery which enables the surgeons to perform the procedure using normal surgical instruments. The table has moving parts to allow the patient to be moved in and out of the MR scanner for intra-operative imaging. Finally, the facility is equipped with a Brainlab VectorVision® Sky neuronavigation system which provides real-time tracking of surgical markers and tools, *global* image registration and visualization facilities. Brainlab also provides image analysis and surgical decision tools (Brainsuite), surgical planning system (iPlan) and other integrated operating room controls. This is illustrated in 1(a).

The current interventional workflow at NHNN acquires iMR images after the temporal pole resection. Using the methodology described here, navigation accuracy for the optic radiation might be improved by acquiring the first set of interventional images right after craniotomy as shown in figure 1(b). This would

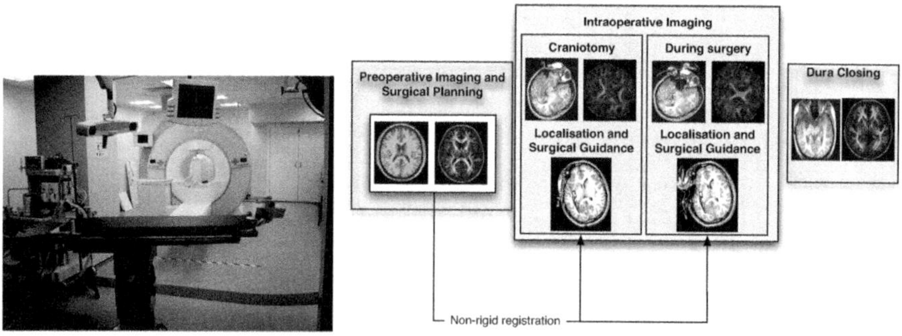

a *b*

Fig. 1. iMR suite with a 1.5T MR scanner and neuronavigation equipment (*a*). Proposed surgical workflow (*b*). The first intraoperative scan is taken right after craniotomy followed by update scans. Images are acquired before closing of the dura to ensure performance assessment of the image guided system.

allow the surgeon to track the target and eloquent brain areas from the onset of surgery and all the surgical plans done on the preoperative images could be brought to the intraoperative space by using fast non-rigid registration. Additional scans could also be acquired during the surgery and the guidance images are updated. Additional images acquired before closing the brain dura would allow continuous assessment of the image guided system on a case-by-case basis by correlating the postoperative patient outcome with the predicted patient outcome at the end of the surgery.

3 Methods

The multivariate NMI measure between two pairs of images $\{R_1, R_2\}$ and $\{F_1, F_2\}$ is given by extending the conventional NMI definition as follows:

$$\mathrm{NMI}(R_1, R_2, F_1(\mathbf{T}), F_2(\mathbf{T})) = \frac{H(R_1, R_2) + H(F_1(\mathbf{T}), F_2(\mathbf{T}))}{H(R_1, R_2, F_1(\mathbf{T}), F_2(\mathbf{T}))}, \quad (1)$$

where $H(R_1, R_2)$ and $H(F_1(\mathbf{T}), F_2(\mathbf{T}))$ are the joint entropies between the two reference images and the two deformed floating images respectively.
$H(R_1, R_2, F_1(\mathbf{T}), F_2(\mathbf{T}))$, is the joint entropy between the four input images and is computed using Shannon's formula for entropy as:

$$H(R_1, R_2, F_1(\mathbf{T}), F_2(\mathbf{T})) = -\frac{1}{N} \sum_{r_1, r_2, f_1, f_2} p(r_1, r_2, f_1, f_2) \times \log(p(r_1, r_2, f_1, f_2)),$$

where r_1, r_2, f_1 and f_2 are the voxel intensity of images R_1, R_2, $F_1(\mathbf{T})$ and $F_2(\mathbf{T})$ respectively.

Each probability is computed using a joint histogram $\mathcal{H}$ as:

$$p(r_1, r_2, f_1, f_2) = \frac{\mathcal{H}(r_1, r_2, f_1, f_2)}{\sum_{r_1, r_2, f_1, f_2} \mathcal{H}(r_1, r_2, f_1, f_2)},$$

where a Parzen Window [8] is used to fill the joint histogram:

$$\mathcal{H}(r_1, r_2, f_1, f_2) = \sum_{\boldsymbol{x} \in R} \left[\beta^3(R_1(\boldsymbol{x}), r_1) \times \beta^3(R_2(\boldsymbol{x}), r_2) \times \beta^3(F_1(\mathbf{T}(\boldsymbol{x})), f_1) \times \beta^3(F_2(\mathbf{T}(\boldsymbol{x})), f_2)\right]$$

where β^3 is a cubic B-Spline kernel.

The similarity measure is maximised using a conjugate gradient scheme and requires the computation of the analytical derivative of the joint histogram which is given by the following:

$$\frac{\partial \mathcal{H}(r_1, r_2, f_1, f_2)}{\partial \mu^{\xi}_{ijk}} = \sum_{\boldsymbol{x} \in R} \beta^3 \left(R_1\left(\boldsymbol{x}\right), r_1\right) \times \beta^3 \left(R_2\left(\boldsymbol{x}\right), r_2\right)$$
$$\times \left(\left.\frac{\partial \beta^3\left(u, f_1\right)}{\partial u}\right|_{u=F_1(\mathbf{T}(\boldsymbol{x}))} \left.\frac{\partial F_1\left(p\right)}{\partial p}\right|_{p=\mathbf{T}(\boldsymbol{x})} \frac{\partial \mathbf{T}(\boldsymbol{x})}{\partial \mu^{\xi}_{ijk}} \right.$$
$$\times \beta^3\left(F_2\left(\mathbf{T}\left(\boldsymbol{x}\right)\right) - f_2\right) + \beta^3\left(F_1\left(\mathbf{T}\left(\boldsymbol{x}\right)\right) - f_1\right)$$
$$\left. \times \left.\frac{\partial \beta^3\left(u, f_2\right)}{\partial u}\right|_{u=F_2(\mathbf{T}(\boldsymbol{x}))} \left.\frac{\partial F_2\left(p\right)}{\partial p}\right|_{p=\mathbf{T}(\boldsymbol{x})} \frac{\partial \mathbf{T}(\boldsymbol{x})}{\partial \mu^{\xi}_{ijk}} \right) \quad (2)$$

The transformation is parameterised using a cubic B-spline model as in [9]. In order to ensure a smooth transformation, the bending energy of the spline is used as a penalty term. We refer the reader to [10] for the computation of the bending energy and its analytical derivative.

4 GPU Implementation

The proposed registration framework achieves parallelism by using the CUDA framework from NVIDIA [11]. Each concurrent thread on the GPU achieves parallel processing by working on independent data. In CUDA, such a GPU function is called a *kernel.* The majority of the GPU kernels for the registration framework are described in [10]. The implementation for the proposed multivariate scheme extends the registration framework to include GPU accelerated computation of the joint histogram and the analytical gradient of the proposed similarity measure.

Computation of the marginal and joint entropies as described in equation (1) is computationally expensive when done serially on a CPU. The core of the computational complexity is shared between the Parzen Window smoothing of the joint histogram and the marginalisation along the target and resampled source image axes to compute the marginal entropies. Considering the use of 64 bins per image, a serial implementation has to perform 4×64^4 iterations in order to smooth the joint histogram. In our parallel implementation, the smoothing of the joint histogram is done on the GPU by using four CUDA kernels; one for each dimension of the joint histogram. For a bin size of 64 along each dimension, we run 64^3 CUDA threads where each concurrent thread effectively smoothes one line of the joint histogram along the given direction.

The marginalisation of the joint histogram along the two target and the two resampled source image axes is split into four CUDA kernels corresponding to each joint histogram axis. Each concurrent thread sums a line along a given direction. To manage loss of accuracy due to the use of single precision floating point in GPUs, *compensated summation* [12] is used for accumulation in these kernels.

The computation of the gradient of the proposed similarity measure is initially computed at the voxel positions using equation (2). This allows each concurrent CUDA thread to process each voxel independently. The gradient at the voxel positions is then convolved with the appropriate cubic B-spline smoothing kernel to extract the gradient at the control point positions.

The source code for the registration framework can be freely downloaded under an open source licence[1].

5 Validation

Numerical Phantom. A numerical phantom was constructed in order to assess the accuracy of the proposed registration framework. For the structural image phantom (see figure 2), a very high resolution digital phantom containing finger and sheet like collapsed sulci and gyri was created, simulating the structure of the cortex. The phantom was created on a 0.25 mm equivalent isotropic image with a size of $180 \times 180 \times 120$ voxels. Gaussian noise was added in the Fourier domain to create the Rician noise corrupted phantom. The fibre tracts were created to span the white matter region of the phantom as shown in figure 2. This phantom allowed for comparison of our proposed registration framework against anatomical or diffusion only registration schemes.

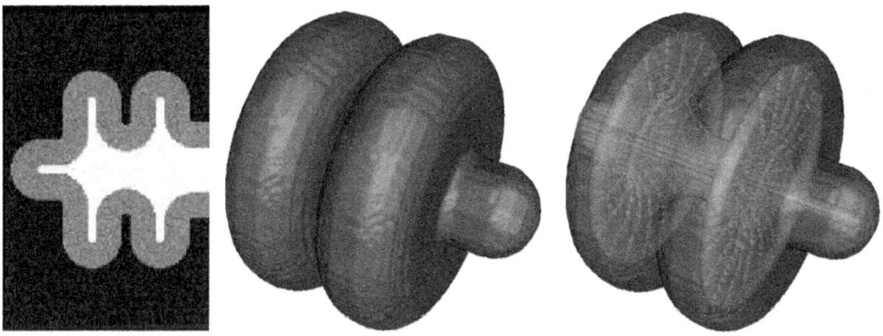

a *b* *c*

Fig. 2. Numerical phantom. (a) shows the simulated cortical layer, (b) shows the 3-dimensional reconstruction of the phantom surface and (c) shows the simulated white matter tracts spanning the phantom.

Known deformations were applied to the phantom and three different registration schemes were used to recover the deformation. First, the structural phantom was registered to the deformed structural phantom to simulate registration between structural images. Secondly, the WM phantom was registered to the deformed WM phantom to simulate registration using the diffusion imaging modality. Finally, we registered the images using our proposed registration framework using the multivariate NMI as the similarity measure which takes information from both the structural and diffusion images. We performed the analysis by repeating the experiment with 100 different deformations. The results over the whole phantom and the white matter area are illustrated in figure 3. Our proposed method improved registration accuracy over the whole phantom

[1] http://sourceforge.net/projects/niftyreg

	Init.	Struct.	Tract	Joint
All	1.69(0.22)	1.15(0.17)	1.50(0.22)	1.05(0.17)
WM	1.70(0.09)	1.08(0.07)	0.92(0.08)	0.87(0.06)

Fig. 3. Mean (standard deviation) Euclidean distance errors in voxels. The second column quantifies the initial misalignment. Subsequent columns correspond to the error after registration using the structural information, the tract information and the joint information respectively. Errors are computed within the whole phantom (All) (middle row) and the white matter (WM) (bottom row).

and also over the simulated white matter regions. Even though the designed numerical phantom is a simple simulation of the temporal lobe environment, it shows that the use of complementary information in a registration scheme can indeed improve accuracy.

Assessment on pre and postoperative datasets. In our previous work [7], we studied 16 patients (8 males, range 17 – 56 years) with medically refractory epilepsy undergoing surgery at NHNN. Informed written consent was obtained from all subjects for this study. The overall aim of the study was to analyse the consequences of surgery for temporal lobe epilepsy. The pre and postoperative datasets were analysed and the preoperatively segmented optic radiation was propagated to the postoperative images. The predicted damage to the optic radiation was quantified and correlated with the measured VFD in the subjects. The proposed method showed a trend towards higher correlation between the predicted optic radiation damage and the subject VFD. The Pearson correlation coefficients for anatomical only, diffusion only and the proposed registration scheme were 0.66, 0.47 and **0.81** respectively. We refer the reader to [7] for a more thorough analysis.

Assessment on iMR datasets. Evidence for improvement of patient outcome must be demonstrated before changes to a clinical workflow can be made. For this purpose intra-operative DTI datasets were acquired from 3 subjects undergoing temporal lobe resection for treatment of refractory focal epilepsy. These data sets were assessed as part of a formal clinical audit exercise according to the data governance protocols at NHNN. In all the 3 cases preoperative T1-weighted MR and diffusion weighted MR data were acquired. Preoperative MR scans were acquired on a 3T MR GE Excite II scanner (General Electric, Waukesha, Milwaukee, WI, USA) and included a T1-weighted coronal volumetric acquisition with a spatial resolution of $0.9 \times 0.9 \times 1.1$ mm. DTI data using 52 gradient directions was acquired using a single-shot spin-echo planar imaging (EPI) sequence with a spatial resolution of $1.9 \times 1.9 \times 2.4$ mm. For all 3 subjects, we also had MR data acquired during the intervention after the temporal pole resection. The intra-operative protocol included a T1-weighted 3D FLASH sequence with TR $= 5.25$ms, TE $= 2.5$ms, flip angle $= 15°$and have a spatial resolution of $1.1 \times 1.1 \times 1.3$mm. DTI data using 30 gradient directions and a spatial resolution of $2.5 \times 2.5 \times 2.7$ mm were also acquired.

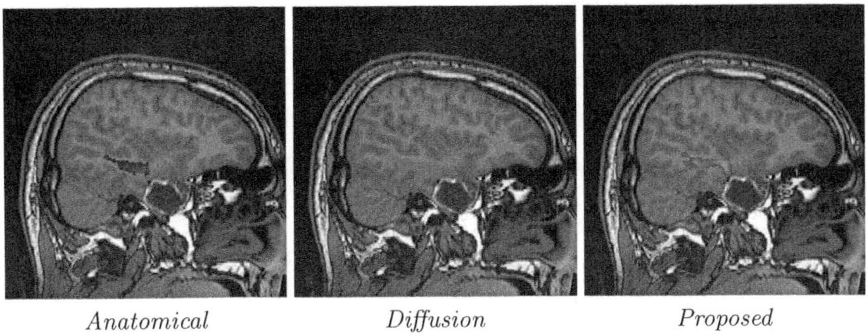

Fig. 4. Subject who showed no postoperative visual field deficit. All three registration schemes show that the optic radiation is intact.

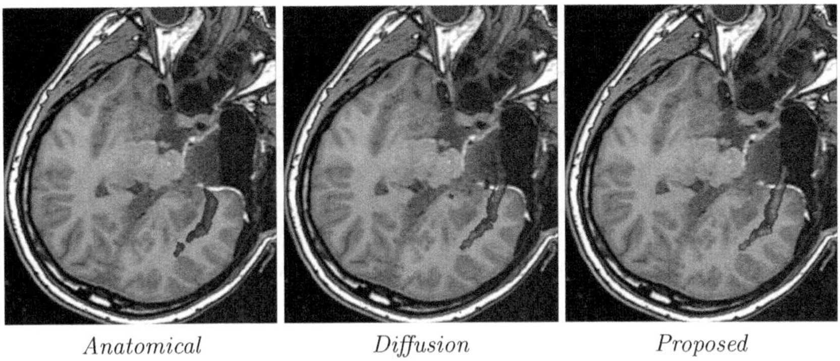

Fig. 5. Subject who showed moderate postoperative visual deficit. The anatomical (red) only registration implies that the optic radiation is currently intact, the diffusion (violet) only and our proposed scheme (green) implies some damage to the optic radiation.

Automatic skull-stripping [13] was performed on the images prior to registration to ensure that non-brain related tissues were removed from the image. The optic radiation was identified in the preoperative diffusion images by performing probabilistic tractography using Camino [14]. A multitensor model was used for the tractography and the probability map was thresholded at 0.05. Three different registrations were performed to map the preoperatively delineated optic radiation to the intraoperative space. Registrations were performed using only anatomical data, only diffusion data using FA images and the proposed scheme which uses both anatomical (T1) and diffusion (FA) images. For the 3 subjects, we show the propagated optic radiation from preoperative to intraoperative space using the three registration scheme. The figures show a selected 2-D slice from this fused 3-D volume for visualisation.

Figure 4 shows the interventional scan for a subject who underwent left temporal lobe resection. The propagated optic radiation using the three registration

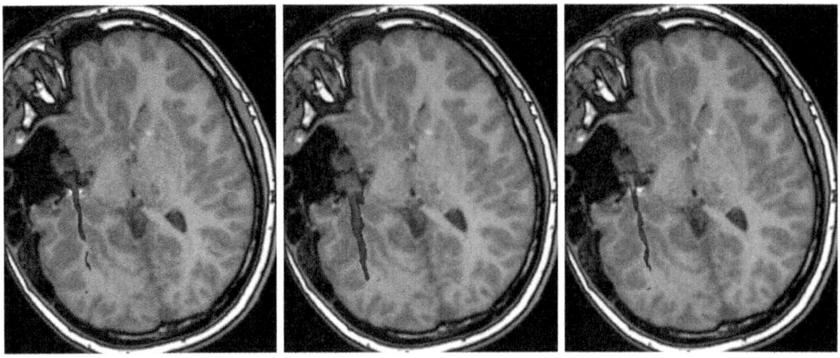

Anatomical *Diffusion* *Proposed*

Fig. 6. Subject who showed severe postoperative visual field deficit. All three registrations show damage to the optic radiation.

schemes is overlaid on top of it. Postoperative assessment showed that the subject suffered no visual field deficit after the surgery. All three registration methods show no damage to the optic radiation. However, the diffusion and the proposed scheme place the optic radiation much closer to the resection than the anatomical only registration scheme.

Figure 5 shows the interventional scan for a subject who underwent left temporal lobe resection. Postoperative assessment showed that the subject suffered moderate visual field deficit after the surgery. The proposed scheme and diffusion only registration shows damage to the optic radiation during the intervention. Anatomical registration shows the optic radiation to be intact.

Figure 6 shows the interventional scan and the localisation of the optic radiation for a subject who suffered a severe visual field deficit after the surgery. All three registration schemes show damage to the anterior portion of the optic radiation.

6 Computation Time

Through the use of the parallel processing capabilities of the GPUs, significant reduction to the computation times were made. We used NVIDIA's C2050 Tesla processors for the benchmarks. The mean time for affine registration of the target and source images for the three interventional subjects was 18 seconds. The average time for non-rigid registration using the proposed method is 2 minutes and 55 seconds. In comparison, the mean time for CPU based affine registration is 37 seconds and for the non-rigid registration it is 25 minutes and 54 seconds. In addition, there is an overhead of doing the skull-stripping and generating the FA images for the interventional scans. However, these times are not significant. The current transfer time of the patient from the scanner to the operating table at NHNN is between $7 - 12$ minutes and the proposed registration framework is fast enough to cope with this time constraint.

7 Discussion

A prerequisite for the effective use of the proposed framework is good quality preoperative and intraoperative imaging data. The limiting constraints for preoperative imaging are less significant and the challenges in terms of image quality assurance lie on the side of the intraoperative image acquisition. The iMR sequence typically used is a single shot echo planar imaging (EPI) due to the rapid speed of acquisition. EPI methods are very prone to geometric distortions due to the static magnetic field inhomogeneities arising from the varied paramagnetic properties of the different anatomical regions especially near tissue-air and tissue-bone interfaces. This can be especially severe for interventional procedures as the resected cavity includes air and can induce high intensity susceptibility. The problem is further amplified by the fact that the wide-bore MR systems often used in intra-operative applications have a smaller uniform static magnetic field region than diagnostic scanners and the subject head usually does not experience a uniform magnetic field as there is limited flexibility with regards to the head placement. Fast correction of MR artefacts like susceptibility would be part of future work. This would enable the creation of a full workflow from acquisition, preprocessing, non-rigid image registration and visualisation that could potentially be deployed in the operating theatre.

8 Conclusion

In this paper we presented a multivariate similarity measure that can exploit the joint information between structural and diffusion images. We formulated the analytical derivative of the similarity measure and incorporated it into a fast registration framework. Parallel computation, through the use of GPUs, has been the enabling technology that makes the non-rigid registration framework feasible for use in a neurosurgical setting. We applied the framework to preoperative and interventional images and demonstrated processing times within the constraints of neurosurgery. Our initial numerical phantom based validation shows improved accuracy of the proposed method over anatomical and diffusion only registration schemes. We applied it to three interventional datasets and the initial trend suggests that there is some variability in the results obtained from the three registration schemes. However, no firm conclusions about the accuracy of the registration methods in the interventional setting can be made from only three datasets and in the absence of a ground truth. Future work would look at a more thorough validation using interventional images that are acquired towards the end of the surgery before the closing of the dura. This would be of use in correlating the localised optical radiation with the postoperative visual field deficit using the three registration schemes and could potentially lead to interesting insights into whether we can achieve the desired accuracy using only anatomical or diffusion images in a non-rigid registration framework or whether, by using joint information, we can substantially increase the registration accuracy.

Acknowledgements

We are grateful to the Big Lottery Fund, Wolfson Trust and Epilepsy Society for supporting the NSE MRI scanner. This work was undertaken at UCLH/UCL who received a proportion of funding from the Department of Healths NIHR Biomedical Research Centres funding scheme. Acquisition of patient scans was funded by a Wellcome Trust Programme Grant (WT083148), Pankaj Daga was funded by EPSRC-CRUK Comprehensive Cancer Imaging Centre of UCL and KCL (grant number C1519AO) and Gavin Winston was funded through a Clinical Research Training Fellowship from the Medical Research Council (MRC grant number G0802012).

References

1. Wiebe, S., et al.: A randomized, controlled trial of surgery for temporal-lobe epilepsy. NEJM 345, 311–318 (2001)
2. Ebeling, U., et al.: Neurosurgical topography of the optic radiation in the temporal lobe. Acta Neurochirurgica 92, 29–36 (1988)
3. Archip, N., et al.: Non-rigid alignment of pre-operative MRI, fMRI, and DT-MRI with intra-operative MRI for enhanced visualization and navigation in image-guided neurosurgery. Neuroimage 35(1), 609–624 (2007)
4. Park, H.J., et al.: Spatial normalization of diffusion tensor MRI using multiple channels. Neuroimage 20(4), 1995–2009 (2003)
5. Avants, B.B., Duda, J.T., Zhang, H., Gee, J.C.: Multivariate normalization with symmetric diffeomorphisms for multivariate studies. In: Ayache, N., Ourselin, S., Maeder, A. (eds.) MICCAI 2007, Part I. LNCS, vol. 4791, pp. 359–366. Springer, Heidelberg (2007)
6. Studholme, C.: Dense feature deformation morphometry: Incorporating DTI data into conventional MRI morphometry. MedIA 12(6), 742–751 (2008)
7. Daga, P., et al.: Integrating structural and diffusion mr information for optic radiation localisation in focal epilepsy patients (2011)
8. Mattes, D., et al.: PET-CT image registration in the chest using free-form deformations. IEEE Trans. Med. Imag. 22, 120–128 (2003)
9. Rueckert, D., et al.: Nonrigid registration using free-form deformations: Application to breast MR images. IEEE TMI 18(8), 712–721 (1999)
10. Modat, M., et al.: Fast free-form deformation using graphics processing units. CMPB 98(3), 278–284 (2010)
11. Nvidia, NVIDIA CUDA Programming Guide (December 2008)
12. Kahan, W.: Pracniques: further remarks on reducing truncation errors. Commun. ACM 8 (1965)
13. Smith, S.M.: Fast robust automated brain extraction. Human Brain Mapping 17(3), 143–155 (2002)
14. Cook, P.A., et al.: Camino: Open-source diffusion-MRI reconstruction and processing. In: ISMRM (2006)

Panorama Ultrasound for Guiding Epidural Anesthesia: A Feasibility Study

Hedyeh Rafii-Tari[1], Purang Abolmaesumi[1], and Robert Rohling[1,2]

[1] Department of Electrical and Computer Engineering
[2] Department of Mechanical Engineering,
University of British Columbia, Vancouver, B.C., Canada
{hedyehr,purang,rohling}@ece.ubc.ca

Abstract. Epidural anesthesia is a common but challenging procedure in obstetrics and surgery, especially for the obese patient. An ultrasound guidance system is proposed using a transducer-mounted camera to create 3D panorama images of the spine relative to markings on the skin. Guidance will include identification of individual vertebrae, and selection of a suitable puncture site, trajectory and depth of needle insertion. This study describes the panorama creation and preliminary testing. The camera tracks the transducer movement using a specialized strip of markers attached to the skin surface, which enables absolute position estimation of the transducer with respect to the patient over the full range of the spine. The 3D panorama image can then be resliced in various parasagittal planes to show either the target epidural spaces or the laminae. The geometric accuracy of the panoramas are validated against an optical tracking system and independent measurements by a sonographer.

Keywords: optical tracking, epidural ultrasound, panorama, guidance, 3D ultrasound, interventional ultrasound.

1 Introduction

Epidural anesthesia involves inserting a needle and catheter into the epidural space between the ligamentum flavum and dura mater covering the spinal cord. The standard method for selecting the puncture site uses palpation of the iliac crest, the C7 vertebra, or the twelfth rib [18]. The correct depth of insertion is determined by feeling the loss of resistance to saline or air injection as the needle tip enters the epidural space. These blind methods are technically challenging, especially for the obese patient, and can result in complications such as dural puncture and nerve injury [10]. The ideal guidance system would provide identification of vertebrae and interspinous gaps, selection of puncture site for desired vertebral level, selection of needle trajectory to intersect the epidural space, and depth estimation along this trajectory from the skin to the epidural space. So far no guidance system has been developed that addresses all of these requirements.

As a safe, low-cost, real-time imaging method, ultrasound (US) has the potential to significantly improve epidural needle guidance by being able to depict

R.H. Taylor and G.-Z. Yang (Eds.): IPCAI 2011, LNCS 6689, pp. 179–189, 2011.

the spinal anatomy and the epidural space [23]. Therefore, we propose a 3D panorama US guidance system with the following specifications: a) Track individual ultrasound images with six degree of freedom with respect to the patient; b) Create a 3D ultrasound panorama from both sides of the spine, using a 2D transducer for its lower cost and simplicity; c) Provide absolute, not relative, tracking with respect to the patient, thereby allowing the transducer to be removed and replaced.

Panoramas are created by reslicing the 3D volume. Two such panoramas are required in this application: (1) a panorama in the parasagittal plane showing the target epidural spaces for trajectory selection, and (2) a panorama in a more lateral sagittal plane, depicting the vertebral laminae with clear interspinous gaps, for identification of the vertebrae. Standard methods of identification by palpation misidentify the spaces in 68% of the cases for the lumbar vertebrae [18]. Previous research has shown that image processing can be applied to ultrasound images to automatically identify the vertebrae [11] and automatically measure the depth of the epidural space [21]. The two different reslice planes mentioned above are needed for these two tasks, therefore a 3D panorama is required. To allow counting from the sacrum, C7, or T12 levels, an extended panorama is needed. Images are obtained from both sides of the spine to enable a complete and clear depiction of the anatomy and the epidural space, given that the spinous processes prevent ultrasound penetration along the midline plane. Absolute positioning is needed because real-time guidance during needle insertion will be performed in the future by replacing the transducer at the desired skin location, determined by analysis of the panorama images.

Since the needle insertion can be performed using a combination of ultrasound guidance and traditional loss-of-resistance [22], the accuracy of the preceding panorama must be sufficient to identify the vertebrae and select an approximate puncture site and trajectory to the epidural space. The accuracy is determined by a combination of factors, such as the measurement accuracy of the interspinous gap location and width, and the identification of the ligamentum flavum (5-6 mm thick [4]). The ligamentum flavum produces the echo defining the posterior aspect of the epidural space, and is the smallest anatomical structure that needs to be identified so that loss of resistance can be performed over the last centimeter of the needle insertion.

It is possible to create a freehand 3D ultrasound panorama solely by processing the image features to detect the relative motion of two consecutive frames, and repeating this estimation over a series of consecutive images [6]. Such "sensorless" approaches are not feasible for the spine, due to complex bone structures resulting in strong spatially-varying shadows and artifacts in the ultrasound image. Conventional systems to explicitly track the ultrasound transducer position are based on electromagnetic, acoustic, mechanical, and optical tracking technologies [15]. Tradeoffs exist among these technologies in terms of range, accuracy, external influences (e.g. line-of-sight and proximity of metal objects) and cost [7]. Optical tracking of the ultrasound transducer location has been performed by many groups with LED's, passive markers, or checkerboard patterns attached to the transducer and/or patient [1,5]. Other approaches have used a combination of local sensors added to the transducer for trajectory reconstruction based on relative translations and absolute orientations with respect to an external frame of reference [20].

With most tracking systems, the position of the transducer is calculated with respect to the fixed external base of the tracker, and then transformed into the coordinate system of the patient, which is also tracked. Movement of the patient is inevitable for this application, especially in the case of parturient patients, because the epidural procedure takes up to five minutes to perform. Direct tracking of ultrasound to skin is preferred. Mounting miniature cameras on the transducer has been previously explored for estimating needle pose and trajectory with respect to the transducer without the need for an external base coordinate system [3,19]. However, absolute position tracking of the transducer with respect to the patient using a single camera mounted on the transducer is novel. By eliminating the external base coordinate system, the tracker range can be greatly reduced, thereby improving the cost and accuracy trade off significantly. This approach also eliminates line-of-sight issues and can accommodate patient motion during scanning.

This paper therefore proposes a low-cost 3D panorama guidance system using a miniature camera attached directly on the transducer and a specialized adhesive marker strip attached on the skin, which allows absolute position estimation of the camera and the transducer over the whole range of the spine with respect to the patient. The use of high-contrast markers is popular for optical tracking in areas of computer vision and augmented reality [24]. The proposed marker is based on checkerboard-like patterns with projective invariant properties, which have been previously explored for pattern recognition and tracking of objects [13,14]. The goal is to provide relatively simple additions to the steps of patient preparation and equipment on a standard ultrasound machine. Although the first intended application is the guidance of the commonly performed epidural needle insertions, other clinical applications are feasible. A similar application is spinal taps where the needle is inserted along the same trajectory but at a deeper depth. Other possible applications include spinal biopsies, regional anesthesia and spinal surgery.

2 Materials and Methods

The implementation of the tracking system involves acquiring standard 2D ultrasound B-mode images, acquiring images of markers attached to the skin using a camera mounted directly on the transducer, determining the pose of the transducer by processing the camera images, combining the ultrasound images and the position data to generate 3D ultrasound panoramas and then visualizing slices of the panorama. Ultrasound images are obtained from the Sonix MDP ultrasound machine (Ultrasonix Medical Corporation, Richmond, BC) using a 5 MHz curvilinear transducer. The Sonix machine is based on PC architecture and contains the SonixRP interface for streaming ultrasound data.

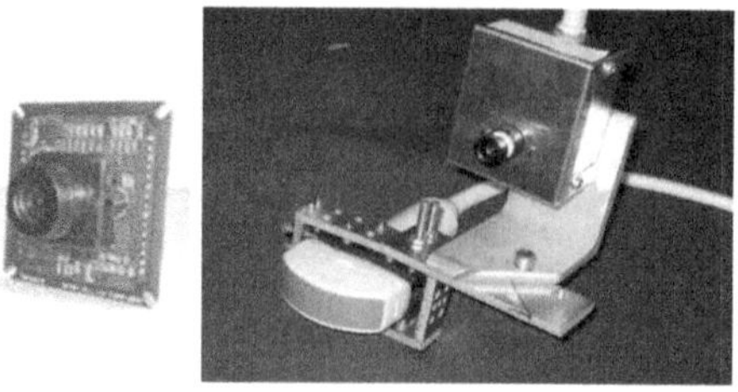

Fig. 1. The ARTCAM-130MI-IR-OP miniature camera, mounted on the transducer

A single ARTRAY-130MI-IR-OP camera is used (ARTRAY Co., Tokyo, Japan). This is a 1/2" CMOS near-infrared miniature camera with a maximum resolution of 1280 × 1024 pixels, a frame rate of 15 FPS and a field of view close to 40 degrees. The camera is mounted on the transducer (Fig. 1), connected to the Sonix machine via USB2.0 and controlled with software implemented on the Sonix. Even though the current apparatus is too large and heavy for routine clinical use, it is sufficient for proof of concept and can be easily miniaturized for future use.

Reconstruction of the 3D freehand panorama was performed with Stradwin [16]. The required steps are camera calibration, marker design, camera image processing and camera-ultrasound calibration.

2.1 Camera Calibration

Camera calibration determines the intrinsic parameters of the camera (focal length, principle center, and distortion vector) using a standard camera calibration toolbox [2]. This is done by acquiring multiple images from different views of a checkerboard and performing a least-squares fit of the camera parameters to match the known checkerboard features.

2.2 Marker Design

The design of the marker uses geometric patterns with unique projective invariant properties. The property of the cross ratio states that if four collinear points (A, B, C, D) are given, the cross ratio can be defined based on the distance between these points according to the following relationship [14]:

$$\text{Cross ratio (A,B,C,D)} = \frac{|AC| \,/\, |BC|}{|AD| \,/\, |BD|}\,. \tag{1}$$

The cross ratio is invariant under perspective projections, meaning that although the relative distances between the projected points change the cross ratio remains constant [13]. Therefore a camera looking at the same pattern from different angles and scales can compute the cross ratio and identify the pattern using only the image coordinates of the four collinear points. The marker design is based on high-contrast checkerboard-like patterns with varying widths and orderings, with

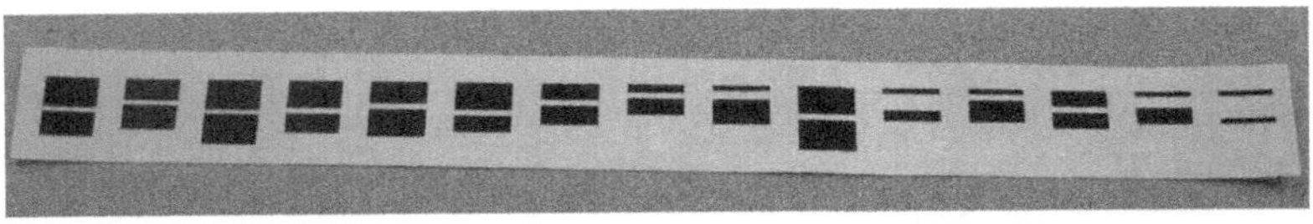

Fig. 2. Marker design with projective invariant pattern properties

each pattern providing four collinear corners on each side, each with a unique cross-ratio. This marker can easily be attached to the skin with the goal of enabling accurate and robust tracking over the whole range of spine. The width of the marker is designed based on the camera's field of view, and the length covers the average length of the spine (approximately 45 cm). The marker strip is shown in Fig. 2.

2.3 Tracking Procedure

The camera images are processed to detect the corners of the patterns, which are found using a Harris corner detector [9]. The detected corners are grouped in four and a collinearity test is performed to detect the ones corresponding to the same pattern. The cross-ratio is then computed to find the position of the pattern on the marker strip by comparing the value to a database containing the minimum and maximum cross ratio values for each pattern, as well as the corresponding 3D coordinates of the corners. Using this information, together with the 2D image coordinates of the corners and the intrinsic parameters of the camera, the pose of the camera is estimated. While this can be performed linearly using at least four coplanar points [17], we choose to use larger number of feature points to improve robustness to measurement errors. For this research, eight feature points and their respective 3D coordinates are used in an iterative algorithm to estimate the pose.

2.4 Calibration of Ultrasound Image

To determine the transformation between the camera coordinates and the coordinates of the ultrasound image, the single-wall technique for calibration is used [15]. A residual error of 1.8 mm was achieved.

2.5 Validation

The accuracy of the overall tracking system is compared to tracking with an Optotrak 3020 (Northern Digital Inc., Waterloo, ON) as the gold standard. Four LED's are attached to the transducer for creating a rigid body to be tracked, and simultaneous camera and Optotrak measurements are acquired. The transformation from this rigid body coordinate system to the ultrasound image is calibrated using the same single-wall technique described above. A residual error of 0.6 mm was achieved.

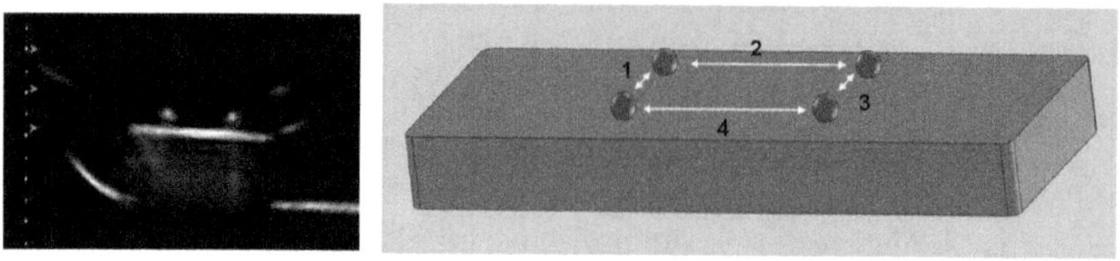

Fig. 3. Ultrasound image of test phantom (left) and four distances measured between beads (right)

The overall accuracy of the panorama reconstruction is evaluated by measuring inter-feature distances of a phantom consisting of a 2×2 matrix (20 mm by 40 mm) of 4.5 mm steel beads embedded in a metal plate, similar to the validation performed in [12]. The phantom with the four inter-bead distances is shown in Fig. 3. The phantom is placed in water heated to approximately $50°C$ to model the speed of sound in tissue. Each bead is imaged eight times at different orientations and depths. The transducer is adjusted until the clearest possible surface reflection is obtained in each image, in order to ensure that the bead is centered in the elevation direction of the ultrasound image. Position measurements for each ultrasound image are obtained from both the camera and Optotrak. The distances between the beads are measured using the Stradwin software by manually selecting the top of the bead in each image, based on the assumption that the sphere surface detected in the ultrasound image corresponds to the top surface of the bead [8]. Using all combinations of the eight observations of each pin gives 64 possible combinations for each pair for each of the four distances, resulting in a total of 256 measurements. The differences between the measurements based on the camera and the Optotrak are calculated.

To test the ability of the system to clearly depict the spinal anatomy and identify the vertebrae *in vivo*, panorama images are created from human subjects (n=4) by moving the transversely-oriented transducer (with the camera attached) in the parasagittal plane, starting from the sacrum. The transducer is moved cephalad on the left side of the spine, then caudad on the right side, with the subject in an upright seated position similar to clinical practice. The marker strip is attached lateral to the spine and is always in clear view of the camera. Camera images are processed to obtain the position information for the ultrasound transducer, and paired to the corresponding ultrasound image using CPU time stamps. The 6-DOF position information obtained from the camera images are smoothed using a moving average filter on a unit quaternion representation, with a span of 11 for each subset of data, and interpolated to match the frame rate of the ultrasound images before being entered into Stradwin.

To confirm the ability of the system for guidance of needle trajectory and depth of insertion, depth measurements from the skin to the ligamentum flavum are obtained from the panoramas for six lumbar and thoracic vertebrae, and are compared to distances obtained from the original ultrasound image at the corresponding levels. The ability to distinguish each vertebra from its neighbours is validated by measuring intervertebral spacings in the panorama, and comparing to measurements made manually by an experienced sonographer for the five lumbar vertebra. Panoramas are registered to the skin by relating the interspinous gaps detected in the panorama to their relative positions on the marker strip, and comparing these to marks made by the sonographer from sacrum to T12.

3 Results

The tests on the phantom showed a 0.9 mm RMS error between camera and Optotrak measurements, with a maximum error of 3.5 mm.

For the human data, panorama images of the spine are created by generating vertical reslices through the created 3D ultrasound volumes. A sample image of the tests *in vivo* is shown in Fig. 4, depicting the lamina for six consecutive vertebrae. Although spine images are obtained from the sacrum up to the mid thoracic levels, the Stradwin software can only depict panoramas up to 1024 pixels at a time, therefore only seven vertebrae are shown in the figure.

Reslices can be created for depicting the ligamentum flavum, which is the last interface encountered by the needle before entering the epidural space. Fig. 5 shows the original 2D ultrasound image, and the reslice panorama depicting the ligamentum flavum at five consecutive levels, confirming the ability of the system for guidance of needle trajectory and depth of insertion.

The depth measurements of the ligamentum flavum at these levels, obtained from the panorama and compared against the depth in the original ultrasound image, show a mean error of 1.13 mm and a standard deviation of 0.68 mm, confirming the ability of the panoramas for estimating the depth of the epidural space.

Fig. 6 shows the levels detected by the sonographer on the left and the reconstructed panorama identifying the sacrum and five lumbar vertebrae on the

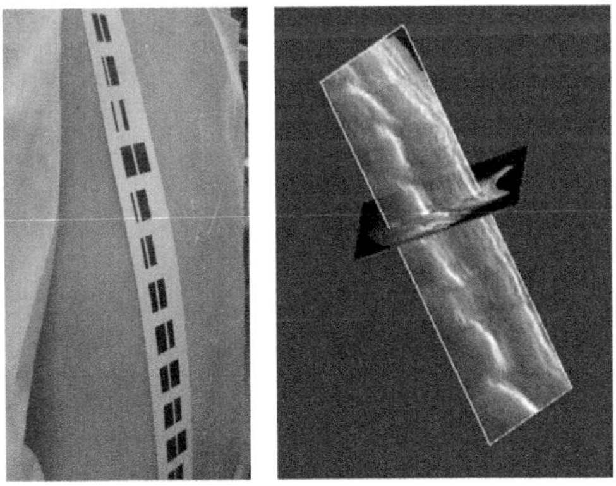

Fig. 4. Marker strip attached to the skin (left) and a portion of the reslice of 3D showing the lamina at six upper lumbar and lower thoracic levels (right).

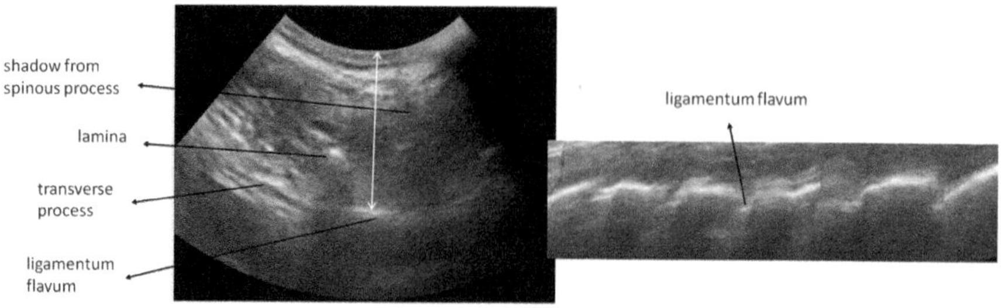

Fig. 5. 2D ultrasound image (transverse plane) and reslice panorama (parasagittal plane), identifying the epidural space from the ligamentum flavum

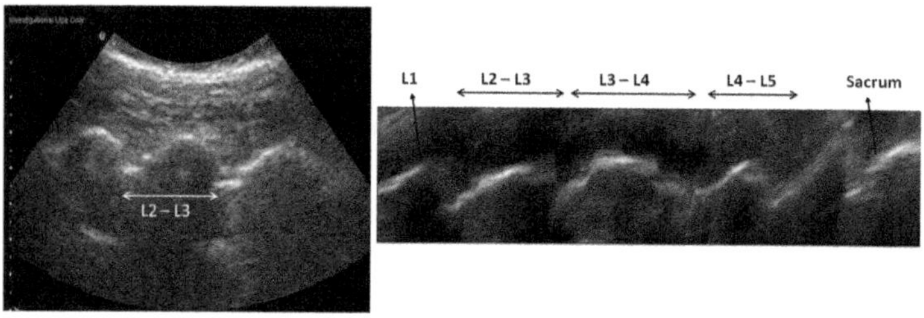

Fig. 6. Standard 2D ultrasound image in parasagittal plane (left) and panorama reslice image showing labeled vertebrae (right)

right, while Table 1 shows the distance measurement obtained by the sonographer against those obtained from the reconstructed panorama in Stradwin. Both the manual measurements by the sonographer and the measurements from the panorama image agree on identifying the largest interspinous distances (L3-L4). The differences between manual and panorama measurements are less than 25% of the actual interspinous distances, suggesting that each vertebra can be distinguished from its neighbour. This is apparent in the panorama image itself, since the lamina of the vertebrae in a parasagittal reslice appear as clearly distinguishable curves.

Table 1. Interspinous distance measurements for lumbar vertebrae

	sonographer measurement(cm)	panorama measurement(cm)	difference(cm)
L4 - L5	2.54	3.14	0.60
L3 - L4	3.32	3.90	0.58
L2 - L3	3.14	3.77	0.63
L1 - L2	2.47	3.07	0.60
T12 - L1	2.56	2.81	0.25

To get an estimate of the variance in the sonographer's measurements, an individual subject was measured repeatedly (L3 - L4, n=10) and the standard deviation of the measurements was 0.83 mm. Given this measure of the sonographer's repeatability, the differences between the panorama measurements and the sonographer's measurements are interpreted to include errors from both the panorama and sonographer's techniques.

The error of registering the panorama to the skin for the six interspinous gaps, compared to marks provided by the sonographer on the marker strip at corresponding positions, was 9.4 mm on average. This average error corresponds to 28% of the interspinous gap, thereby still correctly identifying the levels with respect to the skin.

4 Discussion and Conclusion

The results show that a miniature optical guidance system with a single inexpensive camera and a simple setup can be constructed and calibrated with sufficient accuracy for creating panoramas of the spine, detection of the epidural spaces, and for identification of the vertebrae and the interspinous distances.

The required accuracy for the epidural anesthesia application is divided into several components: identification of the vertebrae, selection of puncture site, and estimation of the depth of needle insertion. The proposed guidance system satisfies the accuracy for identification of the vertebrae (average error is 28% of the interspinous gap), identification of the largest intervertebral space (errors of measuring interspinous gap ranged from 2.5 to 6.3 mm), and depth of needle insertion (average error of 1.13 mm). The 9.4 mm average error for relating the target to the skin means that this technique provides only an approximate puncture site, and that real-time ultrasound guidance should be used for selecting the final puncture site. Note that a change in the puncture site location (e.g. 9.4 mm) has a small effect on the depth of the needle insertion to the target (less than 1 mm based on trigonometry with an average depth of 43.8 mm [21]), but the change in trajectory may produce bone contact. With real-time ultrasound guidance during needle insertion, the bone contact problem is avoided, while retaining the high accuracy of the depth estimation which is the most critical aspect of this procedure to avoid overshoot and nerve damage.

One of the sources of error in the algorithm is the error in the intrinsic calibration of the camera. The effect of this error is estimated by calculating how the standard deviation of errors in each intrinsic parameter can affect the pose estimation of the marker with respect to the camera. The maximum propagated position and orientation errors are 1.9 mm and 0.44 degrees respectively. Other errors arise from extraction of the corner features in the images and estimating the pose of the camera. These are evaluated by obtaining camera images from various parts on the marker strip, using two patterns to estimate the pose of the camera, finding the image plane projections for a third pattern and comparing them to the originally detected corners. The maximum reprojection error is 0.46 mm with an RMS error of 0.15 mm. Another error comes from the calibration between the camera and ultrasound image. The RMS error of the camera calibration is 1.8 mm, compared to an RMS error of 0.6 mm for the Optotrak, showing the greater accuracy of the Optotrak as expected. The cost of the Optotrak compared to the single camera is approximately 100:1. Some error results from interpolating the positions obtained from the camera over all the ultrasound frames. However, given the fast acquisition rate, the change in position and orientation from one frame to the next is very small so the error due to interpolation is insignificant in comparison to other errors.

Future work will involve creating a graphical user interface to display matched panoramas of the spine and skin side-by-side in real-time, with automated ultrasound image analysis to show target, trajectory, and depth of insertion in an effort to increase the ease of use in clinical applications.

The results of this research can have a significant impact on the speed and confidence of the operator performing epidural anesthesia. The next expected clinical application to be investigated with this guidance system is regional anesthesia using needle insertions into the facet joints of the vertebrae.

Acknowledgments. This work is funded by the Natural Sciences and Engineering Research Council. The authors would also like to thank sonographer Victoria A. Lessoway for her assistance.

References

1. Ali, A., Logeswaran, R.: A visual probe localization and calibration system for cost-effective computer-aided 3D ultrasound. Computers in Biology and Medicine 37(8), 1141–1147 (2007)
2. Bouguet, J.Y.: Visual methods for three-dimensional modeling. Ph.D. thesis, California Institute of Technology, Pasadena, CA (1999)
3. Chan, C., Lam, F., Rohling, R.: A needle tracking device for ultrasound guided percutaneous procedures. Ultrasound in Medicine & Biology 31(11), 1469–1483 (2005)
4. Chestnut, D.H.: Obstetric Anesthesia: Principles and Practice. Mosby Inc., St. Louis (2004)
5. Flaccavento, G., Lawrence, P., Rohling, R.: Patient and probe tracking during freehand ultrasound. In: Barillot, C., Haynor, D.R., Hellier, P. (eds.) MICCAI 2004. LNCS, vol. 3217, pp. 585–593. Springer, Heidelberg (2004)
6. Gee, A.H., Housden, R.J., Hassenpflug, P., Treece, G.M., Prager, R.W.: Sensorless freehand 3D ultrasound in real tissue: Speckle decorrelation without fully developed speckle. Medical Image Analysis 10(2), 137–149 (2006)
7. Glossop, N.D.: Advantages of optical compared with electromagnetic tracking. The Journal of Bone and Joint Surgery 91, 23–28 (2009)
8. Hacihaliloglu, I., Abugharbieh, R., Hodgson, A.J., Rohling, R.N.: Bone surface localization in ultrasound using image phase-based features. Ultrasound in Medicine & Biology 35(9), 1475–1487 (2009)
9. Harris, C., Stephens, M.J.: A combined corner and edge detector. In: Fourth Alvey Vision Conference, pp. 147–152 (1988)
10. Horlocker, T.T.: Complications of spinal and epidural anesthesia. Anesthesiology Clinics of North America 18(2), 461–485 (2000)

11. Kerby, B., Rohling, R., Nair, V., Abolmaesumi, P.: Automatic identification of lumbar level with ultrasound. In: IEEE Engineering in Medicine and Biology Society, pp. 2980–2983 (2008)
12. Leotta, D.F.: An efficient calibration method for freehand 3D ultrasound imaging systems. Ultrasound in Medicine & Biology 30(7), 999–1008 (2004)
13. van Liere, R., Mulder, J.D.: Optical tracking using projective invariant marker pattern properties. In: IEEE Virtual Reality, pp. 191–198 (2003)
14. Loaiza, M., Raposo, A.B., Gattass, M.: A novel optical tracking algorithm for point-based projective invariant marker patterns. In: Bebis, G., Boyle, R., Parvin, B., Koracin, D., Paragios, N., Tanveer, S.-M., Ju, T., Liu, Z., Coquillart, S., Cruz-Neira, C., Müller, T., Malzbender, T. (eds.) ISVC 2007, Part I. LNCS, vol. 4841, pp. 160–169. Springer, Heidelberg (2007)
15. Mercier, L., Lang, T., Lindseth, F., Collins, D.L.: A review of calibration techniques for freehand 3-D ultrasound systems. Ultrasound in Medicine & Biology 31(4), 449–471 (2005)
16. Prager, R.W., Gee, A., Berman, L.: Stradx: real-time acquisition and visualization of freehand three-dimensional ultrasound. Medical Image Analysis 3(2), 129–140 (1999)
17. Quan, L., Lan, Z.: Linear n-point camera pose determination. IEEE Transactions on Pattern Analysis and Machine Intelligence 21(8), 774–780 (1999)
18. Reynolds, F.: Logic in the safe practice of spinal anaesthesia. Anaesthesia 55(11), 1045–1046 (2000)
19. Sauer, F., Khamene, A.: Video-assistance for ultrasound guided biopsy. U.S. Patent 6,612,991 (2003)
20. J., P., Stolka, H.-J.K., Choti, M., Boctor, E.M.: Multi-DoF probe trajectory reconstruction with local sensors for 2D-to-3D ultrasound. In: International Symposium on Biomedical Imaging: From Nano to Macro, pp. 316–319 (2010)
21. Tran, D., Rohling, R.N.: Automatic detection of lumbar anatomy in ultrasound images of human subjects. IEEE Transactions on Biomedical Engineering 57, 2248–2256 (2010)
22. Tran, D., Kamani, A., Al-Attas, E., Lessoway, V., Massey, S., Rohling, R.: Single-operator real-time ultrasound-guidance to aim and insert a lumbar epidural needle. Canadian Journal of Anesthesia 57, 313–321 (2010)
23. Tran, D., Kamani, A.A., Lessoway, V.A., Peterson, C., Hor, K.W., Rohling, R.N.: Preinsertion paramedian ultrasound guidance for epidural anesthesia. Anesthesia & Analgesia 109(2), 661–667 (2009)
24. Zhang, X., Fronz, S., Navab, N.: Visual marker detection and decoding in ar systems: A comparative study. In: 1st International Symposium on Mixed and Augmented Reality, pp. 97–106 (2002)

Author Index

Abadie, Alexandre 113
Abolmaesumi, Purang 47, 179
Adebar, Troy 79
Armand, Mehran 36

Balicki, Marcin 55
Bigdelou, Ali 25
Boehm, Andreas 1
Borschneck, Dan 47
Brost, Alexander 133

Cardoso, M. Jorge 168
Carrell, Tom 13

Daga, Pankaj 168
Dastur, Neville 13
Dornheim, Jana 1
Dornheim, Lars 1
Duncan, John S. 168

Echeverri, Santiago 101
Eller, Andrew 90

Fichtinger, Gabor 47

Galeotti, John 90
Gao, Gang 145
Gijsbers, Geert 145
Gill, Jaswinder 145
Goldenberg, Larry 79
Guerrero, Julian 122

Haegelen, Claire 113
Hager, Gregory 55
Hawkes, David 168
Hofmann, Simon 156
Hollis, Ralph 90
Hornegger, Joachim 133

Jannin, Pierre 113

Khallaghi, Siavash 47
Klatzky, Roberta 90
Kwok, Ka-Wai 67

Lalys, Florent 113
Lee, Randy 90
Liao, Rui 133
Lucas, Blake C. 36

Ma, YingLiang 145
Mah, Francis 90
Mahdavi, Sara 79
Mancini, Laura 168
Matthes, Florian 25
McEvoy, Andrew W. 168
Meisner, Eric 55
Micallef, Caroline 168
Modat, Marc 168
Moradi, Mehdi 79
Mousavi, Parvin 47

Navab, Nassir 25
Nguan, Christopher 79, 122
Nolte, Lutz-Peter 101

Oliveira-Santos, Thiago 156
Otake, Yoshito 36
Ourselin, Sebastien 168

Payne, Christopher 67
Penney, Graeme 13
Peterhans, Matthias 156
Preim, Bernhard 1

Rafii-Tari, Hedyeh 179
Razavi, Reza 145
Rhode, Kawal S. 145
Richa, Rogério 55
Rinaldi, C. Aldo 145
Rohling, Robert 122, 179
Rössling, Ivo 1

Salcudean, Septimiu 79, 122
Schneider, Caitlin 122
Schuman, Joel 90
Siegel, Mel 90
Sterner, Tobias 25
Stetten, George 90
Strobel, Norbert 133
Sznitman, Raphael 55

Taylor, Russell H. 36, 55
Thornton, John 168

Varnavas, Andreas 13
Vitiello, Valentina 67

Weber, Stefan 156
Wendler, Thomas 25
White, Mark 168
Wiesner, Stefan 25
Wimmer, Andreas 133
Winston, Gavin 168
Wu, Bing 90

Xie, Weiguo 101

Yang, Guang-Zhong 67
Yousry, Tarek 168

Zheng, Guoyan 101

GPSR Compliance

The European Union's (EU) General Product Safety Regulation (GPSR) is a set of rules that requires consumer products to be safe and our obligations to ensure this.

If you have any concerns about our products, you can contact us on ProductSafety@springernature.com

In case Publisher is established outside the EU, the EU authorized representative is:

Springer Nature Customer Service Center GmbH
Europaplatz 3
69115 Heidelberg, Germany

Batch number: 10844619

Printed by Printforce, the Netherlands